D0457445

Sperm Are from Men,
Eggs Are from Women

"It's been over a quarter of a century since Richard Dawkins's *The Selfish Gene* and nearly a decade since Robert Wright's *The Moral Animal*. It's time for a good update on evolutionary psychology.

"This is not just a good update, it is an approach filled with delight, one that's aimed straight at the heart and soul of your daily life and mine. Joe Quirk's *Sperm Are From Men, Eggs Are From Women,* will reach out and grab the mass audience of *Men Are From Mars, Women Are From Venus* and show them how science can guide them through their lives. Reading it is stealing a treat— snacking on a pastry made specially for you in the private kitchen of a five-star chef."

—**HOWARD BLOOM**, visiting Scholar, Graduate School of Education, New York University, author of *The Lucifer Principle: A Scientific Expedition into the Forces of History* and *Global Brain: The Evolution of Mass Mind from the Big Bang to the 21st Century*

"The factors influencing the mating behavior of the sluts and studs among your hairy-faced ancestors make delectable reading. What's more, these facts are startlingly applicable to your own very present-day meeting and mating behavior. And you thought it was all about personal charm? Joe Quirk's book, *Sperm Are From Men, Eggs Are From Women*, in a most entertaining manner, will let you know differently."

—**ISADORA ALMAN**, Sexologist, columnist of "Ask Isadora," and author of *Doing It: Real People Having Really Good Sex*

"Seamlessly blending science, sex, and humor in his book, *Sperm Are from Men, Eggs Are from Women,* Joe Quirk tempts us with the promise of sexual revelation, and then delivers with an alternately hilarious and astonishing primer on the modern evolutionary theories of human sexual behavior. Quirk's charming combination of corny puns and dry wit leads us, laughing, through what might otherwise be some daunting scientific territory. He plays peek-a-boo with our oldest, most primal urges, triple-dog daring us to confront the possibility that our desires, jealousies, fetishes, and even our deepest emotions are merely the products of our primate past. All who accept the dare will be transformed into scientific thinkers, for observing how we deviate from Quirk's evolutionary stereotypes—and wondering why—is perhaps the most tempting exercise of all."

—**KAREN E. JAMES**, Ph.D., evolutionary & developmental geneticist at The Natural History Museum in London, England.

"Quirk's irreverent, personal style makes learning a lot about sociobiology fun! Expect to be shocked, amazed, disgusted, amused, and in the end, a little wiser about how you approach members of the opposite sex."

—**STEVE M. POTTER**, Ph.D., neuroengineer, inventor of Hybrot, and Professor of Biomedical Engineering at Georgia Institute of Technology

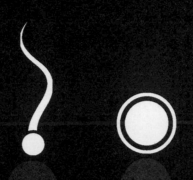

SPERM
ARE FROM
MEN

EGGS
ARE FROM
WOMEN

THE *REAL* REASON MEN AND
WOMEN ARE DIFFERENT

JOE QUIRK

RUNNING PRESS
PHILADELPHIA · LONDON

Library of Congress Control Number: 2005910396

ISBN-13: 978-0-7624-2680-5
ISBN-10: 0-7624-2680-2

Cover and interior design by Doogie Horner
Typography: Bembo and Bulldog

This book may be ordered by mail from the publisher. Please include $2.50 for postage and handling.
But try your bookstore first!

Running Press Book Publishers
125 South Twenty-Second Street
Philadelphia, Pennsylvania 19103-4399

Visit us on the web!
www.runningpress.com

I dedicate this book to Ellen Goodman
for her unconditional support and friendship.

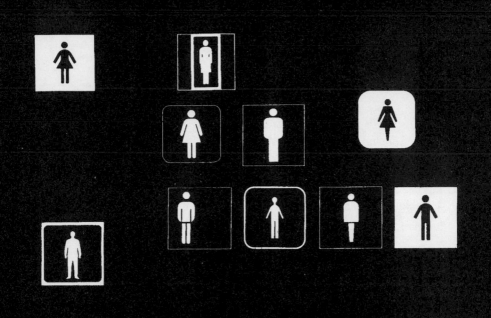

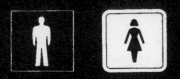

TABLE OF CONTENTS

FORGET MARS AND VENUS.

ASTROLOGY TELLS US NOTHING. BIOLOGY TELLS US EVERYTHING. SPERM ARE FROM MEN. EGGS ARE FROM WOMEN. THAT'S THE REAL REASON MEN AND WOMEN ARE DIFFERENT.

1.

The Sperm and Egg Problem

Why won't he commit? Why does she inexhaustibly want to talk about the relationship? Why can't he finish our first conversation before he's trying to maneuver me into the sack? Why do I have to do so much talking to maneuver her into the sack?

Evolutionary biologists can tell you exactly why. It all comes down to the sperm and the egg. Let's take a closer look at these two troublemakers.

Each man produces one-hundred- to three-hundred-million sperm per ejaculation, or roughly a thousand per heartbeat.

Sperm are worthless. Men are free to waste them, squirt them this way and that. Who cares? There's more where those came from. Half of them come out messed up anyway—broken tails, deformed linings, missing heads. Brainless sperm will try to impregnate a red blood cell like dogs trying to hump your leg. Sperm are not what you would call subtle. There are not many secret mechanisms inside a man designed to gently nurture a sperm. The things just get produced *en masse*, then fired out. Then we make more.

Now consider all the work that goes into producing one egg. An egg is 85,000 times larger than a sperm, a female is born with all the eggs she will ever have, and it takes on average 29.5 days to nurture one precious egg down its silken passageway.

In fact, virtually everything that goes into making a baby is in the egg. The sperm contributes nothing but genetic material. The rest of the sperm is a delivery system, with a few mitochondria carried along as batteries. Picture a submarine crashing into something the size of San Francisco in order to deliver one pizza. The pizza is all San Francisco needs to build something the size of the Earth. The submarine disintegrates into the fallopian sea.

In purely genetic terms, the investment that a *Homo sapiens* male makes in the sex act is a courtship and a few minutes of his favorite thing in the whole world. Then he's free to skedaddle and hope to impregnate somebody else.

Now, think about the genetic investment an Ice Age woman makes in the sex act. She risks nine months of pregnancy, several years of breast-feeding a helpless blob of flesh, then a decade of transforming a rebellious teenager into a self-sufficient adult. At the same time, she has to prevent predators from eating her or her offspring, stave off rapists, and gather enough nuts and berries for two. Plus, she must provide protein for her baby. It ain't easy chasing a woolly mammoth with a toddler strapped to your back.

What we have here are different reproductive agendas. Look at this difference Darwinistically. What would be the optimum breeding strategy for a creature that can produce up to 300 million sperm with each ejaculation?

Spray them around as generously as possible! Sow the fields with them! Shoot, shoot, shoot, shoot! Hurry! One of these darn things has got to take!

What would be the optimum breeding strategy for a creature that produces one egg a month that, if inseminated, requires a lifetime of labor?

Choose wisely.

Look at bison, birds, apes, your dog. Mostly what you see are slutty males and picky females. Males are prancing around saying, "Somebody give me a womb! The more the better!" Females are watching the males display and saying, "Give me one worthy male!"

Spend some time with orangutans. The male fights with other males, shows off to display his genetic fitness, and, if he's lucky, the female chooses him. If she's not lucky, he rapes her. Then he splits. A male orangutan is incapable of feeling love or loneliness, only seasonal horniness. When a female orangutan sees a male, she knows he's after one thing. The child-rearing is all up to the female.

Sigh.

So how did we evolve from monkey business to monogamy? How did we evolve trust from so much lust?

Here's the good news: the amount of male investment in offspring is loosely correlated to the length of childhood dependency. The longer the childhood, the more males evolve toward caring for their offspring.

When an antelope gives birth, childhood lasts about two minutes. The baby antelope reaches a state of self-sufficiency—meaning it can run like heck from predators—almost immediately. It quickly learns how to munch grass and fend for itself. No male antelope care-providers needed.

Imagine if that state of dependence lasted a year. The poor female is trying to protect her helpless offspring from predators all that time. Babies are being eaten left and right.

Further suppose a random genetic mutation in the male antelope causes him to hunt down and bring home grass for his little baby antelope. That male antelope is going to have more descendants who survive to adulthood than all those other deadbeat antelopes. His gene for childrearing will steadily spread through the population.

Let's consider primates. You can draw out a graph and roughly correlate the duration of childhood helplessness with paternal investment. Chimpanzee males provide meat for the females and care for the young for several years. Baboon males invest for less time. Ring-tailed lemur males could care less.

Gibbons are monogamous to the point of piety. The Christian Coalition should adopt as their mascot the white-handed gibbon, with his perfect nuclear family of one loyal gibbette and several gibblets.

Which primate has the longest childhood? *Homo sapiens.* As our brains got bigger, they required early hominid woman to give birth earlier and earlier in the development cycle to fit that huge head out through her cervix. If we gave birth at a stage of brain development comparable to that of normal apes, women would have to be pregnant for 18 months. Which would you rather do, ladies, stay pregnant twice as long and give birth to a toddler's head, or squeeze that kid out a little early? Which will require fewer Pilates classes to change your waddle back to a sashay?

So we pop 'em out earlier. Compared to most mammals, human females give birth to a fetus, and it stays helpless a *very* long time. At the same time, our complicated tribal societies got harder to learn, which favored genes that made childhood longer and longer.

Look at the state we're in now. Our babies won't even be able to breed for more than a decade, and they're not that adept at synthesizing the codes of our increasingly complicated tribes until they're twenty or so. (Twenty-five for my younger brother.)

As our brains got bigger, we had to be born more and more helpless, and our childhoods got longer and longer. Human motherhood became the toughest task in nature.

Meanwhile, there are all these males running around with no genetic investment in their own potential for pregnancy, so their bodies and brains can focus more optimally on other tasks, like hunting baby antelopes. Overworked females can't help noticing they have something these antelope providers want: steady nookie.

I ask you, hominid ladies, which males are you going to have sex with? The males who are sweet and bring meat? Or the males who bail and chase tail?

Males who stuck around raised more offspring to adulthood than males who didn't care. Females who found these loyal males sexy raised more offspring to adulthood than females who found deadbeats sexy. Slowly, dads evolved at the expense of cads.

In many species with long childhoods, female choice bred males to evolve increasing emotional investment in their offspring. Some male birds baby-sit the eggs while the female is off cuckolding them. Devoted deer mice dads raise children who grow faster and survive more often than children of deer mice single moms who raise children Murphy Brown-style. Chimp males offer meat for sex in a kind of courtly prostitution. *Homo sapiens* males offer diamond rings and drive phallic cars to advertise their ability to provide, and *Homo sapiens* females in modern foraging societies unashamedly demand meat from their lovers. Despite the sperm and egg problem that created radically different breeding strategies, our prolonged childhoods meant we evolved to form intense attachments to whomever we happen to be boffing.

Biologists call this the pair-bond. We've institutionalized it as marriage. The bad news is our pair-bond is designed to last for as long as it takes our offspring to reach some level of independence. Genes aren't designed to make us happy. They design *us* to make more copies of themselves. To last "until death do us part," sexual relationships must develop the natural bonds of friendship and affinity that we also evolved on the Pleistocene savanna. How life-long friendship evolved is a subject we will explore later.

But first we have other man/woman problems to tackle, foremost being the differences in what makes male and female hominids horny.

Why do I keep calling you a hominid?

Hominids are all the Neanderthals, australopithecines, *Homo habili*, *Homo erecti*, etc., the upright-walking apes of which we are the only surviving species. Many of these folks roamed the earth at the same time, met, traded goods, possibly mated, and ate each other. Some biologists, along with Plato, define *hominid* as "featherless biped." A hominid is really any extinct ape more closely related to us than the chimpanzee. Our desires, virtues, talents, and demons were developed through their struggles.

Everything unique about *Homo sapiens* brains and bodies was designed on the African savanna during the Pleistocene era. The savanna is an open grassland with clumps of trees. The Pleistocene is an epoch that coincides with the advancement and recession of the last Ice Age, from 1.8 million to 10,000 years ago, when hominids ran amok over the planet, made many large animals extinct—including most other species of hominid—and rapidly turned into us.

Hominids are a subset of apes. Apes are a subset of primates. There are about 235 species of primates, including us.

Monogamous primates tend to be the ones who live in trees. Primates who came down from the trees to compete for ground territory started conniving to hoard mates and sleep around.

When's the last time you slept in a tree? How do you feel about someone walking across your lawn?

A British survey showed that 60% of husbands and 40% of wives admit to cheating on their spouses. The Kinsey Study found that 50% of men and 26% of women under forty in the U.S.A. had extramarital affairs—though *half* of women who read *Cosmopolitan* report infidelities. This is no recent breakdown of family values. These rates have shown no significant changes in a century— except that people are cheating earlier in their marriages.

The problem with surveys is they don't measure how much sleeping around we actually do. They measure how much sleeping around we *say* we do. Humans are notoriously secretive about infidelity, while some tend to exaggerate their conquests.

When I was in high school, my friend Mike Chorost conducted a survey to see how sexually active our classmates were. The surveys were filled out in the bleachers during gym, with much looking over shoulders and giggling. The results were startling. It turned out 99% of boys were having sex with 1% of girls. I was morally outraged! Who were these girls, and why hadn't I been introduced to them? I was tired of being one of only three male virgins in the entire school. I knew the boy figure wasn't exact, though, since I had lied. It also turned out I was the only teenager who had ever masturbated. Good thing I lied about that, too. As I scanned my class of Casanova boys and chaste girls, it dawned on me that the only thing the survey revealed was what we wanted to be true.

Exactly how naughty were we in our ancestral environment? If only prehistoric promiscuity could be precisely measured!

It can.

If you want to know how promiscuous males were on the Pleistocene savanna, look at the size ratio of men to women.

We'll deal with that later.

If you want to know how promiscuous females were on the Pleistocene savanna, look at the size ratio of the male to his testicles.

Let's deal with that right now.

NOTE: Wouldn't you know it, some taxonomists are trying to change the word "hominid" to "hominin" right when my book is coming out. That's because chimps, bonobos, humans, and gorillas were found to be more closely related to each other than they are to orangutans, so taxonomists want a whole new category now. But I'm going to stick with the traditional "hominid," just to annoy them.

2.

Female Promiscuity Controls
the Size of Your Testicles

Psychics gaze into crystal balls and tell you vague things about your future. Biologists gaze at your actual balls and tell you precise things about the scandalous behavior of women in our ancestral past.

Breeding experiments with sheep and mice have illustrated the testicle phenomenon swimmingly. Over the generations, monogamous female mice and sheep have little effect on the size of the males' gonads. But female mice and sheep who are monogamous in public—but promiscuous in secret—quickly cause the evolution of larger gonads in the males.

Let's take a close-up look at your testicles.

First let's measure output. This is no time for squeamishness. When it comes to male ejaculations, biologists take a hands-on approach. The sperm populations of different ejaculates have been measured and quantified. The proof is in the pudding.

Fellahs, you may trust your wife, but your sperm don't. Measurements show that men returning home from a long trip produce a more prodigious amount of sperm—up to 300% more!—for their first copulation with their mates than at any other time. If men see their mates every day, they produce a conservative amount of sperm. The longer the woman is out of sight, the more the male burns extra energy going into sperm production overdrive.

And sperm don't call in reinforcements just to compete with each other. Sperm use teamwork. Many sperm don't try to reach the egg, but fan out in kamikaze blocking maneuvers so comrade sperm can reach the coveted egg. It looks a lot like an American football team blocking for their runners. Get out your microscope and watch these mindless little guys run plays.

Teamwork evolves in nature for one reason: to compete against another team. But where is the other team? Who are these sperm blocking and out-flanking? It's as if the sperm think there is another group of sperm in there.

The scientist's answer: In all apes, testicle-weight as a ratio to male body-weight correlates with the frequency of female "extra-pair copulations."

In English: Male chimps have big balls, because female chimps are big sluts. The second a female goes into heat, she sends signals that no human of propriety would consider decent. She inflames her posterior, douses the whole tribe in scent, and tries to copulate with every male she fancies. Female chimps exercise *some* discrimination, but not a whole heck of a lot compared to a human female. Soon we'll find out why chimpettes defy the standard model of the coy female.

You'd think this would be paradise for the males. Wrong. Every male chimp is a cuckold. Chimp alpha males are in a tizzy, running around trying to stop secret copulations between females and lower-ranking males, but the female drive for sexual variety outwits the male chimps while they are busy fighting. Alphas can only control one or two of these nymphomaniacs—those who throw themselves on other penises every time the alpha male's back is turned—at once. Males can only strategize for a higher percentage of copulations, never for faithfulness. When a chimp female in heat presents her posterior to a male, there could be any number of different guys' sperm already swimming around in there.

This is why primatologists never watch TV. When females go into estrus, the chimp-offs are pure entertainment. It's funny, violent, full of chases and trickery, and it's X-rated—imagine a pornographic *Three Stooges*—and the researchers get to claim that counting erections is scientific research.

But let's recover our scientific *gravitas*. It's not until chimp sperm are analyzed that sexual competition takes on an epic scale. So many gallons of semen go into horny female chimps that the sperm have evolved to work as huge armies. They fan out like S.W.A.T. teams, seek and destroy foreign sperm using chemical warfare, and swim like speedboats toward the egg. Ninety-nine percent of sperm aren't even sperm. They are *anti*-sperm, semen of mass destruction. Inside the chimpanzee vaginal tract, it's a battleground. The sperm fight it out inside her, leaving only a few sperm standing, from which the egg chooses her favorite.

When it comes to the sexual competition of chimps, some of the fight goes on between the big beasts, but most of the battles go on between the sperm. Often it's a war of attrition. The higher your sperm count, the better your reproductive chances. You can believe these chimps are bred for balls.

When the chimp babies are born, nobody knows who is the father of whom, so the male chimps have evolved shared paternity. Female promiscuity pays off in many vaguely-interested fathers. Chimpanzee genes have achieved something human ideology never will—socialist paternity: not much incentive, just a shared half-assed sense of duty.

Remember this scientific principle: The sluttier the females, the bigger the balls.

So where do *Homo sapiens* females fall on the Slut Scale? Let's check the ball barometer of other apes.

Gorillas have teeny, weeny testicles. But they have big shoulders, fangs, and brow ridges. The competition goes on between the big beasts. Sperm can take it easy. There's no selection pressure for them to compete with other sperm, because nobody has sex with an alpha male's female without killing the alpha male. Female gorillas are faithful to the promiscuous alpha male. As a result, gorilla sperm can barely figure out which way to swim. Under the microscope, chimp sperm look like Patton's D-Day, and gorilla sperm look like *Hogan's Heroes*. The male gorilla only gets to mate a couple times a year at most, and his teensy testicles are all he needs to get the job done.

The orangutan male-to-testicle ratio is slightly bigger than the gorilla's to account for the rare instance of a two-timing female orangutan.

Look at you, you big ape. Yes, I'm talking to you, *Homo sapiens* male. What ornaments do you have to distinguish you from a female? Feeble knuckles, slightly more upper body strength, a beard, an ability to read maps, a refusal to use this ability.

Now, look at your testicles. Compared to more monogamous

apes, yours are slightly . . . heftier.

Like your brain. Which co-evolved to impress the big brains of females, which co-evolved to impress your big brain. Everything big on you, *Homo sapiens* male, is big by female choice. Your brain is to wow her with your creations. Your oversized penis—humongous compared to those of other apes—is to please her sexually. Your balls . . . well, your balls are just big enough to suggest that while you were out hunting on the savanna, back on the Pleistocene homestead, women were having a ball.

Rest assured, they don't approach the gigantism of a chimp's. His orgying females have bred his balls to balloon to absurd sizes. Your testicles are one-fourth the body-to-ball ratio of a chimp. But they're four times the body-to-ball ratio of a gorilla. Look at the faithful female gorillas. Look at the promiscuous female chimps. You fall exactly in between.

To produce enough sperm to fertilize a woman, we only need one half of one ball, max. That explains how Benedict Arnold had children. Our balls are an eloquent testament to sneaky hominid women.

Yes, I said sneaky. There is little chance that Pleistocene females attained extra-pair copulations with their mates' permission. The violent jealousy of *Homo sapiens* males is well-established. Psychologist David M. Buss's studies of wife-killing in the U.S.A. and among African tribes found that approximately half were caused by sexual jealousy. In the Sudan, Uganda, and India, sexual jealousy is the leading cause of murder. Worldwide, about 20% of all cases of men murdering men result from rivalry over wives and daughters. Scary stats. Yet hominid females who risked grave consequences to steal a tryst on the side passed on enough genes to be represented in our swollen testicles and paranoid sperm.

You just checked them again, didn't you?

Go on. Feel their weight. Why so much mass to house such microscopic sperm?

I wish there were an alternative theory, but there ain't. Without cheating females, balls just don't get big. Nature doesn't favor organs that require extra energy costs if they don't confer reproductive advantage.

Conduct the test yourself if you don't believe me, *Homo sapiens* male. Next time you ejaculate, grab your microscope. Scientists usually keep one by the bed. (For some reason this doesn't impress the ladies, despite the romantic light emanating from the bedroom Bunsen burner, but if you are a truly rigorous scientist, a bedroom guest is a rare occurrence for you anyway.) Analyze your fresh sample.

You'll notice real sperm don't act like cartoon sperm. Many sperm clasp tails and hold a rear-guard bulwark against intruders for several *days*. To inseminate a female is not just to invest in possible impregnation; it is literally to block her vaginal tract from access by rival sperm. That's why men who have not seen their lovers in a few days can triple their sperm count. This does not happen if the man stays home but just doesn't have sex for a few days. Even if the conscious mind of the homecoming male is assured his mate is faithful, his sperm have never listened to his brain at any time in evolutionary history. Sperm are worried there will be a united front of foreign sperm standing between them and her ovaries, and they arrive in her vagina ready to rumble. Absence makes the heart grow fonder because absence means rivals, and fondness was created by natural selection because fondness resecured ancestral bonds. Still, I wouldn't recommend saying this in a love letter.

Our conclusion? It looks like *Homo sapiens* females evolved in an environment mostly monogamous but, occasionally, females copulated with more than one male on the same day.

Makes you insecure? You were engineered to be insecure, *Homo sapiens* male. Because you have no positive way of knowing that child is yours. Because jealous men passed on more genes. Because males who would rather kill, die, and mete out severe punishments passed on more genes than men who were fine with their mates accepting sperm donations from other men. We even invented a word for such a fool: *cuckold*. There is no verbal corollary for a women who is cheated on. No name of shame.

There is a word for promiscuous women, those wily designers of the testicle: *slut*. There is no corollary for a man who sleeps around. No name of shame. Almost every language in every culture has this double-standard of insults.

Worldwide, the way you insult a male is to tell him his mother is a slut, which is bad. Which means he is a bastard, which is bad. Which means his father was a stud, which is good. In almost all cultures, it's considered good for males to make women sluts, and make their children bastards, but it's bad if your mother is a slut or you are a bastard.

These insult double-standards emerged in almost all languages because of statistical differences in how male and female emotions are structured to protect their genes.

Males of our species should never feel secure in their manhood until men evolve teensy, weensy testicles and disorganized sperm. Our titanic testes are measures of our ancestral cuckoldry.

Next time another male challenges you, "Whatsamatter? Got no balls?" you can answer, "I wish I had less balls."

Whew! I'm glad that seminal chapter is over with. Now let's answer The Great Mystery of the Universe.

3.

What Women Want

I've always envied the male boar. One drop of his saliva makes an ovulating sow become instantly paralyzed in a spread-legged mating posture. No opening line, no expensive dinners, no chit-chat. Just one lick, and boom, she's crazy about you. Talk about a self-esteem boost. Imagine picking out the lady you're attracted to, and guaranteeing your success with an introductory slurp. Maybe Michael Bolton could have pulled it off in his heyday, but most *Homo sapiens* men can only dream of such boarish appeal.

When a *Homo sapiens* male sees healthy young skin, firm breasts, and child-bearing hips, he knows right away that this woman will produce many healthy babies, and he's turned on.

But wait. He also knows he could conceivably impregnate hundreds of such females. Chieftains of the past did it like crazy, passing on their *mack daddy* genes. If all the men in the world dropped dead except that pimply teenager at Kinko's, and women organized a global round-robin to make him repopulate the earth, the young man would heroically shoulder his responsibility to humanity without complaining.

A female would be less excited to be in his position. Anybody who bears the baby is going to want one prime choice for a sperm donor. And the turn-ons are different. A man is attracted to a woman's ability to grow a baby inside her. A woman is attracted to a man's ability to grow a baby outside him. How does he do that? Resources.

Both women's and men's bodies are built to nourish a child on the Pleistocene savanna. One is built to bear and nurse. The other is built to get stuff. In any species that survives by cooperation, stuff is gotten through social power. In all social species with pair-bonds, females are attracted to evidence that males display a chance for power in the community.

Female rhesus macaque monkeys seem pretty good at predicting which males will rise to social dominance. The young low-status males who get extra nookie often grow up to achieve alpha status. There are two ways to interpret this. Either female seductresses magically cause males to become alphas, or female attraction has predictive power.

Why do females have to predict? Why can't females just sleep with today's top dog? It's not so easy when female genes have a split agenda.

Older males with power provide protein. Younger males with vigor promise a future of protection. The two usually don't go together. Older male primates usually have the social standing to control protein markets, yet soon they will get too old to maintain that standing and support their children. Ambitious young upstarts plan to seize power and shift protein-flow to their own children. Females who need protein to assure their future babies' survival have evolved the ability to gauge the potential of young males. Females must size up the ambitious young Turks and ask, "Who will become alpha at his peak and provide my babies with a lifetime of protein and protection?" Female macaque monkeys are attracted to power, but even more so to signs of *potential* power.

The Hillary strategy works more often than the Monica strategy. Any female who's been supplying sex to the new alpha when he was an underdog is sitting pretty. She gets extra meat for herself and her offspring. Her whole family gets status and respect from being associated with a powerful male. If her male gets deposed, status for her and her offspring plummets.

And that's bad. Social standing, to a primate female, can mean life or death. Mothers at the bottom of the hierarchy have trouble feeding their children, and often watch their infants get murdered by other females and males. Mothers on the top of the hierarchy get social support, plenty of food, and even baby-sitting volunteers. Power, to a primate female, means protein and protection for her infants.

Yet it's hard to be a powerful female. Long pregnancy and long infancy means long vulnerability. Power must come through the pair-bond. Among all hierarchical primates, females are attracted to ambitious males.

Humans evolved under these same primate parameters: long infancies, pair-bonds, social hierarchies, pooled resources, complex communication—except multiply the complexity of all those dynamics by twenty. Evolution will favor female primates attracted to prestige and glamour. Did *Homo sapiens* women inherit genes for attraction to high-status men?

Psychologist David M. Buss pulled off a monumental study of over 10,000 people in thirty-seven cultures that revealed amazing consistencies in men's and women's mate preferences. Buss sent researchers to Nigeria, Canada, India, Indonesia, Venezuela, Iran, and many more cultures. They asked men and women to rate eighteen attractive qualities in a potential mate. In all thirty-seven cultures—primitive and modern, monogamous and polygamous, communist and capitalist—women rate prestige and earning power in a potential mate higher than men.

Netherlands women rated financial prospects 36% higher than Netherlands men did. Japanese women rated financial prospects 150% higher than Japanese men did. Women of all other cultures fell between those two. There are no exceptions, even among the obscure Stone-Age tribes: the Tiwi, the Yanomamo, the Ache, and the !Kung. Among hunter-gatherers and technocrats, peasants and aristocrats, Aleuts and Arabs, women agree there's no romance without finance.

In a study of single and married women from Taiwan, Bulgaria, Brazil, the U.S.A., and other nations, females consistently rated "ambition" and "industriousness" as "important" or "indispensable." This was not true for men.

When 1,111 personal ads in the U.S.A. were analyzed, women explicitly specified financial resources eleven times more often than men did. The pattern was clear. Men sought attractiveness and offered resources. Women sought resources and offered attractiveness. An owner of a dating service observed that men look at the photos and women read the resumes. Twenty-something women were the choosiest of all. After that, standards drop, when women claim they grow up and give up on girlish dreams of a knight in shining armor. Well, younger women can afford to have ambitions for a knight in shining armor, because knights in shining armor are competing for them.

In one brutal study, female photos in American high school yearbooks were rated according to attractiveness, then scientists researched whether they married "up" or at all. The results were as you'd expect. Prettiness is a better predictor of the husband's status than the woman's own status, education, or even intelligence. Ouch.

A study of two thousand married women found that those with high-status husbands had more kids, fewer divorces, and rated their marriages as happier. Psychology experiments demonstrated that women strongly prefer ugly guys with Rolexes over handsome guys in Burger King uniforms. (That does it. I'm never going on a date in sweatpants again.)

But remember, a woman needs a Pleistocene provider for fifteen years at least, so it doesn't do her much good to marry the 70-year-old chief of the tribe. The Anna Nicole Smith strategy could be a problem if the old chief kicks off while she's breast feeding and a new chief inherits his status. Women must predict future chiefs, so women are less attracted to power than ambition for future power. Girls in fairy tales hung their hopes not on the king, but the prince. Remember guys, the car you drive is not as sexy as how driven you are.

When a man makes a million, it has an attraction effect like when a woman gets breast implants. If these mate preferences were the product of cultural conditioning, we would find cultures where older, high-status women marry young, nubile males, and young, nubile males are seducing older, high-status women. There are none.

Nobody is saying all women cynically marry men for money. Women really do fall in love. Women really do get horny.

But if our feelings are sincere, our genes are Machiavellian. Watch any fifty-year-old male professor dating some college cheerleader, and you know men's emotions are structured to fall for mere fertility. But why is she dating him? Did genes structure female emotions to fall for mere signs of prestige? If only human communication contained some subliminal message as to what women want from $ex and what men expect to get from financial sucksex.

First we'll analyze my personal research into what makes heteros horny.

Then we'll find out why love turns us into idiots.

Then we'll find out why idiots in love are the smartest people alive, though they're too stupid to know it.

4.

Bodies and Resumés: What Makes Us Horny

Let's look at some of my fan mail. Let's see . . .

"By what authority do you pontificate about the 'biological' differences in men's and women's behavior, you sexist?"

You'd be amazed how often I am asked this question. I crashed a scientist's party in Berkeley and rapidly started winning or at least sabotaging every debate I got into. Soon, I was surrounded by Ph.D.s. I was insisting that the human genome is analogous to a novel, in that it is a linear digital alphabet whose code creates life. I pushed my pomposity to sublime heights. I had just finished B.S.ing my way through the helix structure when some smart-aleck post-doc asked if I had any credentials.

Uh . . . credentials?

No, I'm just some guy. I studied literature and minored in

Development of Western Civilization at Providence College, taught partially by Dominican priests who had no sense of humor when it came to my biological observations about celibacy. I graduated at the top of the bottom tenth of my class. That may not seem like such a big accomplishment to certain Ph.D. scientists, but among *my friends*, I was the brain. I attended one year of law school before I was kicked out for smartass-ery, so I only lost one third of my soul, which is just enough to function in a capitalist economy. I invested the last seven years of my novel royalties in reading evolutionary biology studies, full-time. Now finally I feel ready to ask a woman on a date.

Me and schools never got along. Education interferes with learning. I'm an independent scholar, a Renaissance man, a free thinker. Okay, fine, I don't have any qualifications. I live in Berkeley, so I can challenge intellectuals to debate and pray they don't ask me if I have any credentials.

Besides, I've done direct scientific research. Yet when I tell people that I bend over backward to study sexuality, they laugh.

During my thoroughly unromantic days as a struggling novelist, I had occasion to work minimum wage as a light and sound technician for a one-night-only fashion showcase for men's clothing. There were only females in the audience. I was not invited to model. I had to provide spectacular light shows and dope beats, while male hunks strutted the stage in various wardrobes. Casual wear. Out about town. Winterwear. The women acted like scientists: frowning in puzzlement, sighing unromantically, the occasional yawn. The swimsuit strut got some scattered giggles, especially the thong that displayed serious cheekage. But mostly it was lively as a lab room in there. My lights and music weren't adding any spice.

Then these guys marched out in power suits.

The women went ape. I witnessed something approaching a simultaneous group orgasm that lasted about five minutes. The stage was partially rushed. People ignored the fire lane regulations. I'm talking senior matrons acting like schoolgirls at an *NSYNC concert. Purse items were thrown. Was I going to have to call the riot police?

I was confused. How could putting on some stupid clothes be more sexy than the actual butt-thonged guy?

Ever the rigorous scientist, I quickly checked this behavior against my other research in the field.

I've attended bachelor parties. (Purely as a scientific experiment.) I found that male arousal correlates precisely with stages of female disrobal. I measured these findings by jaw slackitude, paucity of eyeblinks, length of tongue-waggliness, and the impulse to yell "woo" in a feminine falsetto—very similar to the mating cry of the Siamang gibbon. I discovered that the eye-goggliosity ratio was inversely proportional to the correct use of syntax, indicating a rapid flow of blood away from the higher neocortex brain functions toward some as-yet unknown organ. Further scientific measurements became untenable as I got distracted. I had to attend many such events to cross-check my findings. I feel ready to present the scientific community with my theory.

What was happening here? Men were responding to displays of genetic fitness as manifested in bodies. Women were responding to displays of genetic fitness as manifested in symbols of status.

I concluded, late in life, as most men do, that if you want to impress the ladies, maybe putting on some nice clothes isn't so stupid.

And I'm losing the thong.

5.

Why Men Are Afraid of Commitment, Women Cautious about Consummation

A fertile woman in her underwear. It's arousing. It's arousing because men see her fertility.

A fertile man in his underwear. It's funny. It's funny because women see a man stripped of his status displays.

Granted, this report could contain a sex bias. It takes discipline as a primate with a gender to write about fellow primates and maintain your scientific objectivity. In fact, some scientists are known to betray their gender in the way they phrase their scientific reports.

I define male *Homo sapiens* as strong, patient, reasonable, and tolerant, while female *Homo sapiens* are soft, pliable, creamy, and wrong. Can two such radically different creatures ever understand each other as objectively as we scientists?

Since long before the time of Socrates, philosophers have puzzled over the Great Questions of Life: Sex is fun, so why don't women offer it indiscriminately? Committed intimacy is the deepest human need, so why are men so terrified of it? Luckily we have evolutionary biologists around to get these Pleistocene puzzlers squared away. The source of our conflicts is in our genes, and the secret to compromise is in our genes. How to make love stay? Listen up.

Guys, gals, stop trying to figure out what's going on in your mate's brain. Skip that part. We'll never get anywhere with the brain. I'm going to write a whole different book about that. First think about their genes, which designed the brain.

Reproductively, each gender has a tremendous gift to offer. That gift is easily exploited, thus extreme emotions evolved to defend it. You'll notice each gender tends to be touchy about certain issues. So let's all just settle down, take a deep breath, put on our lab coats, peer into a Petri dish, and ponder the zipper structure of each other's chromosomes. There. Have you stopped thinking about sex? Can we get scientific please? Thank you. Now, unzip each other's genes. What do you see?

A woman's tremendous reproductive gift is her womb. Much of her food energy goes into maintaining this complicated apparatus. If a sperm gets in there, and it takes, to chicks, that's a big deal.

A man's tremendous reproductive gift is the resources he can acquire because he doesn't have a womb. He can put his food energy into upper body strength and throwing talents, because he must invest a lifetime of work into a child he can't be sure is his. If somebody else's sperm gets into his mate's womb, and it takes, to dudes, that's a big deal.

Everybody's emotions are structured to protect the great reproductive gift of their gender.

Female genes know sex doesn't just mean some enjoyable experience. Pregnancy means resources and work and little time to acquire more prestigious sperm. Choosing to have sex severely limits the reproductive potential of a womb-protector.

Male genes know commitment doesn't just mean some emotional experience. Commitment means resources and work and little time to shoot sperm into other wombs. Choosing a pair-bond severely limits the reproductive potential of a sperm-spreader.

If a woman gets pregnant in the Pleistocene era, and the father high-tails it for the hills, her babies can die. The babies she could have had with another mate if she had never met the deadbeat might never get conceived.

If a man invests a lifetime of work into his Pleistocene mate, and her offspring is not his, his babies might never get conceived. If he finds out, all sorts of people can die.

Next time your mate is having a spaz, remember his or her genes, and try to be patient. His commitaphobia, workaholism, jealousy, and obsession with breasts and sports—it's all for the children. Her teasing, PMS, vanity, and obsession with glamour and shoes—it's all for the children. When you think of male and female "stereotypes" as glandular reflexes genetically designed to protect our future children, we can cut each other a little more slack. If you think the emotional weaponry designed to protect unborn children is extreme, just wait until they're born.

Unfortunately everybody's emotions are also structured to exploit the gift of the other sex. Any valuable biological gift you have is also a weakness that can be taken advantage of. We may choose to be upstanding and honest. But our emotions were structured by the ruthless logic of natural selection. Your genes don't stop at tricking your loved ones. They trick you, too. Now let's figure out their secrets and trick them back.

Male *Homo sapiens* find it easy to act like potential husbands in their quest for sex. Once they get sex, often they are surprised to find their feelings change. After all, each man has enough sperm for every womb in the tribe. Natural selection gave man a penis and a brain, but only enough blood to run one at a time.

Female emotions are structured to exploit this blood-flow problem. Females of many pair-bond species are attracted to stable males who possess resources. Females of these species are also attracted to risky males who have "bad boy" genes that can be passed on to virile offspring. These are two different types of attraction.

If you make sperm, and childhoods are long, centuries of Darwinian selection will split your reproductive interests into two strategies: quantity and quality. One emphasizes baby-making, the other baby-rearing. Emotions for both strategies exist in every man, because every man is the descendant of hominids who made extra surviving babies using both strategies. Every man has a dad and a cad in his genes.

If you have a womb, and childhoods are long, centuries of Darwinian selection will split your reproductive interests into two strategies with different goals: resources and genes. The two don't always come in the same male. The best resources might come from your husband. The best genes might come from somebody else's husband. Emotions for both strategies exist in every woman, because every woman is the descendant of hominids who made extra surviving babies using both strategies. Every woman has a wife and a concubine in her genes.

Emotions are instincts, instincts come from natural and sexual selection, and you can see Pleistocene dynamics in our fears. Women are afraid of being abandoned. Men are afraid of being trapped. Women are afraid men will invest labor in some other woman's babies. Men are afraid to invest labor in some other man's babies. Sperm-spreaders and baby-bearers have inherited a different suite of fears and urges from the Pleistocene savanna.

This is the key to the dual mating strategies in the genes of all animals with long childhoods, which we will explain next chapter. Once we understand the desperate dynamics that created our Pleistocene emotions, males and females will understand each other better. Then evolutionary biology will tell us how we fall in love and stay loving. Then we will get to gay love, an astounding way that nature found to copy genes.

First let's get to good girls and bad girls, good boys and bad boys, and all the babies they made.

6.

A Do-It-Yourself Home Experiment

Before we get to that, first conduct this do-it-yourself home experiment: have sex. You'll need a colleague. Your body should come with the proper kit. If you are a womb-carrier, execute the experiment your normal way. If you are a sperm-spreader, immediately after orgasm, scream, jump up, dash out the door, and speed away in your car. (Wait, for some guys, that *is* the normal way.)

Now analyze how you feel. If you are a womb-protector, my years of scientific research gives me power to predict that you will feel tricked. You wanted something good you didn't get. If you are a sperm-spreader, you should feel like you got away with something. You got something good for free.

Now conduct Phase Two of the experiment: *pretend* you want to have sex. Increase your ardor, then change your mind at the last minute. Tell your partner you have too much respect for this new pair-bond to cheapen it with early sex.

If you are a sperm-spreader, my way-too-many years of research have taught me the hard way that you will feel tricked. You wanted something good you didn't get. You've put a lot of energy into this without getting anything back. Who knows if you will ever get it.

If you are a womb-protector, you should feel honored by this gesture. You got something good without giving up something. You should also feel absolute power to veto this gesture, and decide that, actually, now is the time. The difference in these two reactions is the key to the evolutionary roots of our desires.

7.

How Men Get Sex

You can't just rank a man's sexiness by his salary. Lots of wealthy CEOs can't get a date. Money didn't even exist a million years ago. The real Pleistocene currency by which a hunter was ranked was not cash but attention.

Through all of *Homo erectus* and most of *Homo sapiens* evolution, tribes were semi-nomadic, and the material wealth you could amass amounted to what you could carry—or what you could make other people carry. Hominids still displayed their expensive possessions— before SUVs there were seashell necklaces—but what they really wanted was respect. How much crap you owned was less important than how many people wanted to do you a favor. The real natural environment of hominids was less the savanna than the social group. If you were a hominid male, and people paid attention to you, craved your approval, shut up and listened when you spoke, that meant you were a leader. Men who commanded attention commanded access to community support. That meant a good nest-maker.

Our nests weren't permanent, but moved across the landscape. We humans were less homesteaders than campers. That's why human nests are less material than social. Look at all those other hominids in your community. They're your real nest. Most of the crap we accumulate is a structure to impress them.

Humans compete less for territory than for rank. Territory and possessions are only symbols of rank. The attention of the tribe is a kind of psychic territory where we harvest the resources we cooperative apes need to survive. He who controls the attention is high status and sexually attractive.

That's why rock stars get more than CEOs. The bullet points on your resume don't elicit the same visceral Pleistocene reaction as fame.

And it helps to be a male professional basketball player. That means you combine the five big fitness indicators that get a heterosexual woman's ovaries singing: height, fame, wealth, body symmetry, and athleticism. You're going to have trouble scheduling time to play basketball.

But those of us who are short, unknown, poor, lopsided klutzes shouldn't give up hope. Susan Blackmore, who wrote *The Meme Machine,* says that for 2.5 million years, women mated with the best spreaders of *ideas*. That's why today, women might prefer an ugly broke guy if the tribe incorporates his ideas. Bullshitters get the babes? I read that, and I started writing this book. Shoot *this* through a hoop, Jordan.

I don't care whether you are a primate or a pipefish, all social systems among animals are hierarchical. Our ancestral tribal societies were economically unequal. A whole lot of hominids were competing for a small number of high-status positions in the tribe. This means only a few ended up on top, a few on the bottom, and the rest somewhere in the middle. We inherited their desire to be popular, their sexual attraction to popularity, as well as the pretense that we are too good to care about popularity. The human race is a race.

Now we know how men get sex. Can we guess how women catch men? Did women inherit any instinct to compete for attention?

Let's conduct an anthropological study of the modern dating scene and measure how much single women angelically nurture each other.

8.

The Catfight Gene

Among species that don't have pair-bonds, female sexual jealousy does not exist. What's the point of fighting over a male? Orangutan females would rather fight over food, which at least has some value. After they have sex with a male, he is free to chase whomever he wants. What do females care? They only wanted his sperm, and there's plenty to share. Let the males fight amongst themselves, the girl orangutans think. Whoever comes out on top has the best genes, and we'll all get some. Orangutan females would make terrible contestants on *Elimidate*.

When pair-bonds do exist, however, as with many birds and some mammals, females compete viciously to secure long-term bonds with males.

I've seen elegant bridesmaids claw each other's faces when the bouquet takes to the air. *America's Funniest Home Videos* has as many clips featuring body-checking for the bouquet as they have clips featuring blows to the balls. What is wrong with these spazzes?

The Ache tribe of Paraguay is aptly named. One third of their children die before they are fifteen. If you're born among the Ache and you have a dad, there is a 20% chance you will die. If you don't have a dad, there is a 45% chance you will die. Father absence triples the probability of death by disease or bad diet, and it doubles the chances that the child will be murdered or sold into slavery. Anthropologists have found all sorts of abstruse ways to say what needs to be said plainly: When food is short and children are at stake, people suck.

But the Ache don't ache any worse than other tribes who still live as our ancestors did. Across all hunter-gatherer societies, 20% to 65% of children die. Now you know where you get your extreme feelings concerning romantic matters. Love feels like a matter of life or death, because it once was. We inherited ancient aches.

A tribe is like the *Titanic*. When things start to sink, wealth and privilege decide who lives and who dies. Everybody wants to marry up, to the upper decks where the lifeboats are.

Now imagine that you're the gender who gets so pregnant you can't run, who gives birth to a plump ball of fresh baby that can be smelled from miles away, who must load that baby up with protein for fifteen years before it can breed for itself, and who has a body that invests more calories in womb maintenance than muscles useful for killing. What's going to be important to you? A lifelong bond with a loyal hunter/warrior who will protect your community and provide for your family at any cost. Contrary to the popular bumper sticker, fish need bicycles. (Some fish prefer fish, but lesbian love will be explained later.)

Women want paternal investment as much as men want paternity assurance, and women will fight dirty for it. There has always been severe selection pressure for females to be sexually attracted to signs that predict fatherly investment and signs that predict leadership power. And there are only a limited number of leaders.

Fifteen-year-olds among the Ache are not children. They are hardened adults who carry weapons and bear children and know damn well what's important: popularity, power, pair-bonds, paternity assurance, paternal investment, and protection of kin through threat of violence. These six P's keep your babies fed. Every famine, somebody's kids have to starve, and the only way the powerful make sure it isn't their kids is to claim extra. Yet nobody will survive without wide-scale cooperation. This is the bind that explains lots of our social emotions.

Of course, nowadays this correlation between status and offspring is thrown out of whack. Once we *Homo sapiens* kicked off the industrial revolution and passed out contraceptives, farm food, and vaccines, the poor started breeding much faster than the rich. But, among modern hunter-gatherers—and for almost two million years of the Pleistocene epoch during which our desires evolved—the prestigious produced more surviving children. The environmental dynamics that created our emotions have changed, but the emotions have not.

We don't need to look at hunter-gatherers to find evidence that popularity made our ancestors happy and horny. We can look at agricultural societies just before the industrial revolution. During the 19th century, Swedish villages kept precise records of birthdays, marriage dates, number of children, and occupations as if they had a modern bureaucracy to help them. Anthropologist Bobbi S. Low wrote a book called *Why Sex Matters: A Darwinian*

Look at Human Behavior, and her graph of 19th century Swedish birth rates as correlated to wealth is sobering.

Wealthier women usually had twice as many births at every age as the same number of poor women. And this just measures fertility rates—it doesn't even include stats on who survived childhood because of better nutrition. Likewise, richer men had more chance of remarrying and producing more offspring. Bobbi Low shows how in every generation, the less ambitious, less successful, and less fortunate were breeding less, while the more ambitious, successful, and fortunate were breeding more. Even though we're talking about Swedish villagers whose lives were much less harsh than those of the Ache, in every generation, there was selection for genes for greed and status-grubbing, as well as genes for sexual attraction to the greedy and popular. This explains why Robin Leach has never hosted *Lifestyles of the Broke and Obscure*.

Status competition is the furnace in which our species was forged. There is a stubborn social hierarchy among humans, and the cavewoman who mates with the most socially powerful male raises the most secure children.

This is why she needs a real diamond engagement ring, not a fake one, and why it doesn't matter if she can't tell the difference. A woman does not love a diamond ring because it is sparkly. If that were true, a rhinestone would do. A woman loves a diamond ring because of what it symbolizes: a man promising to nest-invest. If it ain't expensive, you ain't investing.

That's why a feminist ideology can't convince most bridesmaids they don't need men any more than an educated neocortex can tell them that thrown bouquet is just a stupid symbol, so why should I even bother to—*wait, did that bitch just push me?*

9.

The Jerk Gene

Any male hominid can, in theory, impregnate every female in the tribe. But resources are scarce. Twenty flings that result in ten children won't help your genes much if all those children starve or are born in low-status positions in the tribe. Any random genetic mutations that caused males to focus their resources on one female and her babies would get passed on as more of those babies survived to adulthood.

But, hey, it can't hurt to throw a few extra sperm out there. After all, the world is full of wombs. There's no big investment for the male in mere sex. Offspring he raises and offspring he leaves to chance don't have to come from the same womb. Just because *Homo sapiens* males have evolved deep bonding with their offspring and mates doesn't mean they don't have, deep in their limbic systems, primal memories of the ancient male slut strategy. Sluttiness is always the default strategy of any sperm-maker.

Most male animals pursue a "quantity" strategy: inseminate as many females as you possibly can and leave the offspring to chance. This usually causes vicious competition among adult males.

Among 115 bull elephant seals studied by zoologist Burney LeBoeuf and others, five of the biggest and meanest warriors sired 85% of the offspring. Ninety percent of bull seals die virgins—yet even those who reign for one spring of war and orgy are dead by the next year, so wounded are they from their brief season of glory.

You may laugh at the weird-looking platypus, but you wouldn't do it to his duck-billed face. The same number of males and females are born. Then male juveniles start killing each other with poisonous spines. By the time that generation is ready to mate, there are 6 females for every male. These victorious and polygynous warriors then sire a new generation of bad-ass platypi.

Other male animals develop a "quality" strategy: produce a few choice offspring and stick around to make sure they grow to become breeders themselves. This tones down male-male competition considerably, because they're too busy fathering. In general, the more males father, the less they fight.

The male red fox is a devoted husband and dad. (I'm talking about the animal, not the actor.) He brings home a dead rabbit every six hours, teaches the kids how to stalk and hunt. He even buries food to teach his pups how to sniff it out. But if a young foxette in heat slinks by, it's not like the male red fox doesn't notice. Foxes, like us, are serially monogamous.

The Djungarian hamster from Mongolia is a dedicated father. He harvests the land, stuffs seeds in his pouches, scurries back to his burrow, stands before his pups, then hits his cheeks with both forepaws to spray the seeds all over them, just like John Belushi with his zit joke in *Animal House*. Pop does the same trick when he acts as midwife for his mate, slapping her cheeks with his forepaws. It's hard to tell if she appreciates this, and it doesn't cause the same pop-out effect, but it's the effort that counts. If Pop meets another female on a business trip however, this rodent might act like a rat.

Unfortunately for marital relations, genes for an overriding "quality" strategy will never entirely select against a "quantity" strategy in any organism that produces millions of sperm. No matter how much hard work a male invests in his offspring to assure their survival and status, he always has spare sperm. When your sperm is like Old Faithful, it's harder to be faithful. Comedian Chris Rock said, "A man is only as faithful as his options."

This means men will inherit two different kinds of sexual desire, because men make two different kinds of children: Children they invest in, and children they abandon. Children of wives and children of concubines.

Some men impregnate out of lust, then look in their hearts, and are surprised to find they don't feel any deep compulsion except the one to run away. The same men will get somebody pregnant out of love, and they will work their lives away for that wife and family. Men don't necessarily plan this cynically. The reproductive history of their sex rewarded them with two strategies: pair-bonding and sperm-spreading, so evolution will pass on two different kinds of feelings to them.

Women will be less likely to experience this bifurcation. A baby comes from your body, plain and simple, and it doesn't matter whether the father is a saint or a shit-heel. You don't have extra eggs to toss around, and you can't attach the kid to your husband's breast while you go out with your buddies.

A researcher asked people about the minimum intelligence level they would require of a potential date. On average, both men and women said average intelligence. And how intelligent would the date have to be just to have sex with them, asked the surveyors. The women said, well, in that case, above average intelligence. The men said, well, in that case, below average intelligence.

Even among *Homo sapiens* with our prolonged childhoods, male feelings will be structured to love the primary mate and children, but still be capable of supplemental sex without emotional commitment. Over the millennia, male *Homo sapiens* evolve to look at some women as potential wives, others as potential concubines. Women's concern that they are still "respected" after sex suddenly sounds like their genes asking, "Am I a potential wife or concubine?"

This is the female bind. Women know that to entice men, sexual behavior is necessary. Yet they also know that if men perceive them as promiscuous, they may put them in the concubine category and not the wife category. A man's desire to assure paternity means he is less inclined to invest his resources in a woman who is promiscuous.

Freud analyzed men's madonna/whore complex thusly: "Where they love they cannot desire; where they desire they cannot love."

Well, it's not *that* bad, Sigmund. Men feel lust and love for the same woman all the time, but only when she embodies a man's two reproductive goals: baby-birthing bodies and baby-rearing behaviors. Good bodies and good mothers don't always go together, which is why every man has a playboy and a father in his genes. Good genes and good fathers don't always come in the same man, which is why every woman has a concubine and a wife in her genes. Many women make healthy babies with the concubine strategy, but the wife strategy has been more successful. Otherwise, the female preference for wife status would not have evolved.

But it's the twenty-first century! you're saying. Women have demonstrated their power to earn great prestige alongside the most powerful men! Why should the high-earning bad-ass babes of the modern age care about some man's earning power?

Amazingly, Buss cites several studies that independently demonstrate that high-earning women in the U.S.A. are even more demanding in their desire for status in men. Female millionaires want male billionaires. B.J. Ellis showed that even leaders of feminist organizations demand wealthy men as mates. Jackie Kennedy and Princess Diana, moving on from royalty, bedded billionaires. Cleopatra famously had trouble finding a guy who was good enough. When you're literally considered a goddess, only an emperor will do—and even that's a step down. It's hard to marry up when you're the woman on top, but top women keep trying.

Every predator's favorite prey is the helpless young. Our young stay young a long time. Our most primal emotions were structured when men and women were vividly aware of this fact. That's why no matter how much we can logically deduce that highly-paid women armed with diaphragms don't need men's help, our deep Pleistocene need for companionship will always be part of human nature. Whether or not we need each other practically, we will always need each other emotionally.

I know there's plenty to eat. You know there's plenty to eat. But our mammalian limbic systems, which structure our desires, remember that when famine hits, the young die first while the powerful get the spoils.

And whichever sex gets the spoils, spoils it for the other sex.

When men have power over resources and the moral codes of their society, they surround themselves with harems of extra wombs. What happens when women get the power? Guys, imagine the precise opposite of your porno fantasy, then go visit the Bakweri of Cameroon, and see how closely it matches up.

The West African Bakweri babes of Cameroon run a feminist utopia that is a man's dystopia. Mass emigration and immigration can wreak havoc on your society's gender balance. Among the Bakweri, there are 2.5 men for every woman. Women own the plantations and hoard all the money. Yet women do not keep stables of young, nubile men to fulfill their sexual whims. Nor do they create a benevolent Earth Mother society of sharing and socialism. Instead, they demand disposable husbands from the small proportion of men who have resources, and divorce them as soon as they've sucked them dry and a richer fellow is available. Bakweri women treat men as work horses, and unashamedly cite economic ineptitude as the reason for divorce.

In fifty cultures where inadequate earning is a sanctioned reason for divorce, forty-nine of them allow only the woman to initiate divorce. In one, either husband or wife could initiate divorce for economic incompetence. No culture allows only a man to divorce his wife because she's a bad provider. Yet the concept of men sharing their resources with women is a human universal.

According to Nancy Etcoff's article in *News Digest*, anthropologist Suzanne Frayser surveyed divorced people in forty-eight traditional cultures. One of the top two reasons for divorce cited by women was that the man was a bad provider. The number one reason cited by men was infertility (typically blamed on the woman).

Interestingly, Bakweri women's economic power does not

liberate them from prostitution. Hey, it's a seller's market in Cameroon. Many single Bakweri women amass a sizable treasury for themselves by charging exorbitant sums for sexual services to desperate men. By the time they are ready to marry, these entrepreneurettes have fistfuls of cash and acres of property, and they are ready to claim their first husband and bleed him dry, black widow-style. Fortunately, she stops short of feeding him to her offspring—though my girlfriend sometimes looks at me like she'd consider it.

Normally, I'd stop and take a rest here, but I better keep writing to stay one step ahead of my competitors. Mornings I work on this book, but nights I switch over to my great work of literary art. I have this deep inner calling. . . .

10.

Bower Birds Teach Us How Art Evolved to Get the Groupie

Why do artists long to make art? Why is art useless, and why do we sanctify it? Evolutionary biologists say art evolved for courtship. Let's take a look at that womanizer of the art world, the male bower bird.

Each male bower bird builds a gigantic Taj Mahal hundreds of times his own weight for no other purpose than to coax females inside for three seconds of sex. Tall enough for a human to enter, colored with so much flower pulp, butterfly wings, and berries, these nests rise out of the drab forest like hallucinations; these woven cathedrals put a whole new spin on the concept of "love nest." Some species even add lawns of green moss, or avenues and promenades leading up to the palace gate. While strutting, singing,

and tap-dancing around their masterpieces, male bower birds van-
dalize each other's bowers as in some romantic comedy.

Females arrive to play art critic. Symmetry and color coordination are very important to them, just as, in the sideshow of male
bower bird ballet, symmetry and body coordination have the most
aesthetic appeal. Females make their judgments and step inside a
bower.

Boom! The show is all the foreplay they get. And forget cuddling.
No sooner do males mate than they get right back to strutting
for the next groupie, while the female hurries off to build an efficient teacup-sized nest in which to brood over her eggs and raise
her chicks as a single mom.

Could our elevated taste in art have evolved for the same
beastly purpose? Many evolutionary biologists think so. Genes for
the urge to create masterpieces would get favored in our ancestral
environment if humans found artists sexually attractive. The theory
of sexual selection proposes that early men and women must have
kept choosing to mate with creative people because creativity displayed genetic fitness.

And this is the sexiest idea in evolution. The greatest force
in evolution is our turn-ons. Our need to hunt down caribou
and forage for berries evolves us much more slowly than whom
we choose to sleep with. Our environment built us to run,
breathe, eat, squat, throw things, dig for tubers, and find shelter.
But men and women bred each other to be smart, creative, witty,
loyal, and beautiful. Through the eons, we built our own bodies
and minds through our mate choices. Organisms are self-creat-
ing. Next time you decide to sleep with someone, remember the
whole species is at stake. If you have sex with a jerk, you're
selecting for jerk genes.

To understand why mate choice evolves us much faster than natural selection, you must understand the difference between natural selection and sexual selection.

Natural selection evolves organisms to solve problems in nature. Sexual selection evolves organisms to impress members of the opposite sex. It's easy to tell them apart.

First, natural selection. Adaptations designed by natural selection to solve problems in nature are cheap in energy cost, efficient, and specialized. There is very little variety among members of the same species, because natural selection weeds out less efficient adaptations. Natural selection hones every trait for optimum efficiency, to get the job done with no extra frills. It causes all the Spartan beauty of organisms: a cheetah's form, a frog's fingers, an eagle's wingspan, a mosquito's brain, a kangaroo's perfect kidney.

Natural selection also emerges in an organism's behavior: eating, sleeping, locomotion, flatulence.

Now, sexual selection. Adaptations designed by sexual selection to impress mates must be ostentatious, the more wasteful the better, and pointless except to impress. There is wild variety within species, because each member is trying to distinguish himself from a reproductive competitor. It's where all an organism's baroque showoff-y beauty comes from: a lion's mane, a toucan's colors, a daffodil's flowers, a warthog's warts, a human's unnecessarily humongous breasts and penises.

Sexual selection also emerges in an organism's behavior: a rooster's strut, a bower bird's architecture, a frog's burp, an amateur's biology book.

When you see a lion chase down a wildebeest, you're seeing qualities and behaviors honed by natural selection. When you see the male lion furrow his mane and stick out his chest, and the female lioness slink onto her back and raise her tail coyly in the air, you're seeing qualities and behaviors created by sexual selection.

Sexual selection changes organisms much faster than natural selection, because the inanimate environment doesn't care whom it selects, whereas a horny animal cares very much whom it selects. The trials and tribulations of cruel nature weed us out much more slowly than the trials and tribulations of trying to find a date.

Now we know why Picasso got so many chicks. Ever see a photo of Picasso? Not exactly Robert Redford. Nor was he the snazziest dresser. But he could make one hell of a bower, and he knew how to strut and dance around it. He talked the talk. Art is less grandeur than grandstanding.

Ladies, next time your guy complains about taking you out to a fancy dinner, remind him that if he were the Australian golden bower bird, he'd build you a giant structure over sixty feet tall, and weighing several tons, with nothing but his feet and beak.

If your man ever *does* build a sixty-foot structure for sex though—and it's made out of orchids, snail shells, regurgitated fruit, and shingles stolen from your neighbor's house—worry that he's done bower bird research and found out that the male bower bird never has to do a lick of work once pregnancy is achieved.

Makes you look at Trump Towers in a new light, doesn't it?

Art is like the twitter of the chickadee: a display of mental fitness, a form of sexual ornamentation. Good singers get the groupies, whether they are male or female, cock or bushtit. Music and plumage get you sex. No wonder Gene Simmons is named Gene.

Female sexual ornamentation is rare in nature, but it occurs in two instances: when the females are promiscuous and must compete with each other for males, or when species are monogamous and both males and females must impress each other.

Whoever doesn't compete for a mate ends up drab. Whoever has to compete for a mate gets to be fancy. A monogamous female seabird, the crested auklet *Aethia cristatella*, has a large crest to show off her health to males.

The exciting thing about our species is that women evolved sexual advertisements just as males did, including artistic creativity. This means both hominid men and women had to compete for Pleistocene mates. Without competition among same-sex rivals, there's no reason to grow various breast designs or beards or build bridges or win at bridge.

Hey, I like to make art for art's sake, too. We don't work to succeed in order to make more babies, but we inherited genes for the urge to succeed because it used to make more babies. Humans work for reproductive currency, whether we know it or not. What, do you think I'm writing this for the advancement of science? I learned early that the only reason men do anything is for women.

When I was twelve, my Boy Scout troop arranged for a week-long trip to a Canadian island. No females allowed. Many of our fathers were strict. They approved of our scouting because it would teach us discipline. Yet the moment we arrived on our isolated island, fathers gave up bathing, shaving, raising children, and moving muscles for the whole week, while we boys were free to create our little Lord-of-the-Flies society, complete with face paint and ganging up on fat kids. I was mystified at how these once noble patriarchs couldn't seem to muster the energy to get out of their hammocks or brush the crumbs off their bellies. Their only orders involved delivery of food, booze, and water, in that order. One of them demanded we dig a latrine within drunken-stumbling distance of his hammock. I couldn't understand why he didn't just move his hammock closer to the latrine we already had dug. Back home, my father used to punish me for not keeping my fingernails clean, yet on our island I felt free to light underbrush on fire; blow up bee's nests with gasoline; chop down trees with axes; play chicken with motorboats; play "manhunt" barefoot in the middle of the night; chase human prey through poison ivy; jump off 40-foot cliffs into the shallow water; drink Jack Daniels; vomit; and allow my inevitable pocketknife cuts to become infected and pus-filled. It wasn't until day six when it was time to go back to the world of women that our fathers dragged themselves out of their hammocks, used some soap, changed their shirts, sobered up, and ordered us to scrub the six days' worth of fly-ridden pots. And let's see about getting those leeches off your back so Mother doesn't see.

Men may be the man of the house, but women rule the roost. I was a professional nanny for five years. (Hey, you try being an unpublished novelist.) I was intimately involved with several dozen families, and though I never made a scientific study, I can make a sweeping generalization about dads and moms that never had one exception. When it comes to children, women rule with an iron hand. Fathers have about as much clue as to what's going on as they had when they were courting their wives.

This is what happened if I got a dad on the phone:

"Hello?"

"Hey, this is Joe. I was wondering what time Maurice needs his medicine."

"Uhhh . . . well, my wife is not here, so—"

"Do you know if he got it at breakfast? It says here on the bottle every four hours—"

"Well, uh, we always make decisions together, and I don't want to get in trouble."

"Okay, do you know if I have to pick up Clarice? Because if I do, you'll have to come get Maurice. And bring Zelda or he'll have a fit."

"I have a kid named Zelda now?"

"Zelda, his favorite stuffed animal. Can you do it?"

"Uhhhh, well, I'm not allowed to leave until she gets back, so—"

"Okay, do you know when she's coming back?"

"She didn't leave instructions."

"Can you take a message for me?"

"Uhhh, I'm not sure."

"What do you mean, you're not sure?"

"There's no pen here."

This is what happened if I got his wife on the phone:

"Mom speaking."

"Hi, this is—"

"I'm glad you called! I gave Maurice his medicine at 8:20 in the car to time it so he gets his next dose at 12:20 as he's finishing his lunch. I stapled an automatic alarm to his lunch bag to remind you. You'll need to put gas in the car after, not before, you drop off Maurice. It's going to get overcast mid-day, so he needs his blue jacket for recess, and his karate uniform for karate. Clarice is still upset about what her friend Jane said to Jill about Joanna concerning the boy she likes, so I need you to tell her she's pretty at 3:15 on the way to band camp where she'll see Joanna. I set the dashboard alarm to remind you."

"I think I need to write all this down."

"I already did. It's pinned to the phone you're holding."

Moms never check with Dads before they issue their edicts.

Moms memorize their kids schedules down to five-minute incre-
ments and know the names of all their friends—imaginary or
otherwise. Dads can't even keep the goldfish straight. Moms are so on
the ball, dads don't even try to compete and consider themselves
lucky if they can follow orders.

Why do men make worse mothers than women do? Because
sperm-makers specialize in sex and violence.

11.

Male Promiscuity Decides Your Height

Polygyny is sex with multiple females. Polyandry is sex with multiple males. Polygamy is just extra sex in general.

Among mammals, the bigger the males are than the females, the more polygynous they are.

Gibbons are mostly monogamous, and males and females are the same size.

Alpha male gorillas control harems of as many as six females, and are double the weight of each female.

The southern elephant seal male averages a harem of fifty females, and weighs, typically, nine times as much as the diminutive seven-hundred-pound females.

The correlation is perfect because of male bullying.

The more females one male can monopolize, the more other

males die celibate, and so the fiercer the competition for wombs. As the biggest and strongest always get to breed, genes for size and strength in the male are continually favored in the population until you end up with the gigantic male elephant seal.

Remember, lady mammals: The bigger the males, the bigger the harems.

Perhaps by this point our lady readers have developed a scientific curiosity as to where *Homo sapiens* males fall on the Slut Scale.

Homo sapiens males are on average 8% taller, 20% heavier than the females. A biologist seeing such a difference in another species would casually conclude that the males of this species are mostly monogamous but mildly polygynous.

Oh, stop acting so surprised.

Among mammals, polygynous males almost exclusively do rough-and-tumble play. Little males wrestle to practice for future dominance bouts to hoard mates.

Monogamous male mammals like the California mouse don't wrestle much. They are too upstanding for such nonsense. The only female mammals that engage in rough-and-tumble play are carnivores. Among all other mammals studied, the youngsters engaged in the most vigorous rough-and-tumble play are polygynous males.

Do our little males show this mate-hoarding behavior?

I still remember my own kindergarten "nap time." Girls pretended to nap. Boys wrestled. Beginning at age three, boys engage in much more rough-and-tumble play than girls. By age four, boys hit, push, and trip—which they define as "just playing"—almost five times more often than girls.

Also, did you ever notice how awkward an eleven-year-old boy looks dancing with an eleven-year-old girl? His face is at breast height, yet he's too immature to appreciate it.

The late sexual maturity of males of other mammals is related to how much they have to duel with each other for mates. Polygynous males mature late, because they need more time to build up the big plumage or antlers or fangs or muscles to compete. Before they sexually mature, males and females of most species look alot alike—basically like mom. It's not until puberty strikes that males start sprouting fancy accoutrements. The more you fight to hog mates, the later you mature.

Northern elephant seal females mature by age three, whereas males are mature at age eight. Male satin bower birds mature at age seven, and females mature in half that time. That represents some serious ancestral male fighting. In our species, boys don't reach puberty until an average of two years after girls. The sudden pubertal growth spurt in boys follows the same pattern as that of other non-monogamous primates. This speaks of an evolutionary history of some males fighting for extra mates, while other males get none.

Without some polygamy, sex differences do not evolve. In species of perfect monogamy, males and females evolve most of the same qualities. Male and female gibbons, those paragons of monogamy, are hard to tell apart. Even many ornithologists can't tell a female swan from a male swan until they capture them and stick a magnifying glass between their legs.

Promiscuity causes what biologists call "sexual dimorphism," meaning males and females look different. The promiscuous sex usually has the most extravagant traits. Male ducks are fancy because they're studly. Male gorillas control lots of mates, and they have great crests on their heads, giant fangs, huge shoulders, and big brow ridges. The male gorillas smart enough to survive to advanced years have silver backs.

Remember this scientific principle: the faithful sex looks drab, and the slutty sex looks fab.

Pretend you're a biologist from outer space studying the sexual ornaments of *Homo sapiens*. Males have facial hair. Females have oversized breasts. Males have oversized penises. Females have exaggerated waist-to-hip ratios. Looks like somebody in our ancestral past was getting a little nookie on the side. The striking fact that both sexes have sexual ornaments tells us both sexes had to compete for mates. And both sexes had some power of mate choice.

But differences in sexual ornaments in general only give you a base. You've got to check the main sexual ornament, what biologists call "the primary fitness indicator" of the species. This is your sexiest quality. These are the peacock's tails, the bright bellies of female pipefishes, the extravagant qualities which are the most honest advertisers of an animal's health and the biggest turn-ons to the opposite sex. Though men's and women's "secondary sexual advertisements"—breasts, beards, buttocks—are very different, our "primary fitness indicator" is almost identical between women and men.

Homo sapiens' "primary fitness indicator" is our brains. This is because, in our species, brain power counts for much more on the reproductive front than size.

Homo sapiens' intelligence is not attached exclusively to the male, as a peacock's tail is attached exclusively to the male. The remarkable cognitive similarities in men and women show that hominid males and females had a roughly equal ability to breed each other for intelligence.

Nonetheless we do have one or two cognitive differences. Women are better at keeping track of many things in space. Men are better able to turn shapes around in their heads and still recognize them. This is because women gathered and men hunted. Females had to remember where edible plants were and keep track of toddlers. Males had to chase game past hills and trees, and then remember how to get back when all his landmarks were backward and in reverse order. Men focus and women multi-task.

These separate skills inform flirtation. When it comes to the courtship device of our brains, women can juggle many balls at once, while men don't beat around the bush.

Lay out all these variables on your graph for *Homo sapiens*: Male and female average difference in mass is 20%. Males mature on average about 20% later than females. Body ornaments are extravagantly different. Behavior is mostly alike (with some note-worthy statistical differences) especially in aggression levels. Cognitive abilities are almost identical, with a few differences which will fascinate us in later chapters and explain everything we ever wanted to know about that weird other sex.

Put it next to your graph for other primates. Judging by the Slut Scale, *Homo sapiens* males have evolved in conditions far more monogamous than those two-timing male gorillas, orangutans, and chimps. But we are significantly less monogamous than our more distant relatives, the gibbons.

Maybe it's unfair for us to leap to the conclusion that men are all a bunch of slavering dogs. Our polygynous traits might be resid-ual evolutionary leftovers, like your appendix, your tonsils, and your canine teeth. Maybe australopithecine guys were doing all the bul-lying and messing around, and *Homo sapiens* men are on a steady evolutionary shrink as their muscle fiber adjusts to their moral fiber. After all, the loudest barkers of family values are men, whose urge to strut and shout might not be related to their secret urges. We should judge modern men not by how biology structures males, but by how men structure cultures.

An ethnographic survey of 849 societies revealed 16% are

monogamous, 83.5% have men with multiple wives, meaning polygynous, and less than one-half of a percent are polyandrous, which means women have multiple husbands. In all polygynous cultures, men declare themselves moral leaders.

But not all the men in polygynous societies get to have extra wives. There aren't enough females for that. In polygynous societies, 60% of marriages are monogamous. Most of the remaining husbands can afford two wives. It's only the wealthiest men who get three or more wives. This means that in five out of six modern societies, wealthy men monopolize most of the wives, and low-status men die bachelors.

Looking back in time, polygyny is even more pronounced. Almost 1,000 of the 1,154 past or present societies studied allowed a man to have more than one wife. That's close to 90%.

Polygyny is not just a non-Western phenomenon. Jews practiced it until Christians told them they couldn't in the Middle Ages. Christians practiced it through the Middle Ages almost as much as their priests. And why shouldn't they? The Old Testament is so chock full of polygyny it's hard to keep the genealogies straight. Our founding fathers practiced polygyny with their slaves like Old Testament kings. Polygyny in the U.S.A. was legal until a little more than a century ago, but some Mormons still practice it anyway. When I heard this, I told the nearest Mormon I was ready to convert, until he mentioned that I had to support every wife and child on my writer's income, plus wear that outfit. Now we know why Mormon males make so many sacrifices for their faith.

Polygyny for the powerful was the pattern throughout our species' evolution. All of us are the descendants of powerful and promiscuous men who were rewarded with extra descendants, which means all men inherit genes for ambition and promiscuity, and females inherit genes for attraction to ambition and promiscuity.

Donald Trump. Babe Ruth. Henry Kissinger. Not one of these guys would make it as a Calvin Klein model. Yet they are all notorious for womanizing. Martha Stewart, Margaret Thatcher, Indira Gandhi, and other powerful women do so little man-izing there isn't even a word for it. Thanks to evolution, sperm-shooters and womb-protectors have different desires.

Despite the evolution of the long-term pair-bond, we may safely conclude that the mostly monogamous *Homo sapiens* males did some double diddling. We are all the descendants of bastards.

Thus we inherited various needs.

Next time you see a group of naked *Homo sapiens*, look at them as a biologist for once. You can see that men's bodies specialize in mating, and women's bodies specialize in parenting. We can see this same specialization in the bodies and behaviors of most species. Consider the big differences between males and females in most species:

Males make low parental investment. Females make high parental investment. Males can potentially make thousands of babies. Females can potentially make a few. Males show high levels of sexual activity. Females show lower levels of sexual activity. Males do most of the competing. Females do most of the selecting. The more females impregnated, the better it is for the male's genes. The better the male selected, the better it is for the female's genes.

Motherhood is much older than fatherhood. Fatherhood is the male's imitation of the ancient female instinct to nurture offspring. Males of most species are interested primarily in sex, and could care less about their offspring—if they even know who their offspring is. It ain't easy getting a sperm-maker to behave like a parent. How did female hominids manage to breed males to be so fatherly?

For sensitive male attachment, we have to thank the mystery of menstruation.

12.

Why Women Are Coy, Men Clueless

Blame secret ovulation. That's where the confusion started.

Homo sapiens males became more like female mammals in general in that they developed long-term bonds with their offspring.

Homo sapiens females became more like male mammals in general in that they got hornier.

Yes, hornier. Most female mammals are chaste all through their cycle. Then suddenly, for the few days they are ovulating, female mammals go through a Jekyll-and-Hyde transformation. They go into estrus. "Estrus" means the female grows a giant sign that says, "Me so horny." In apes, it's usually a giant pink butt, or an aphrodisiac aroma, or the tendency for the female to stick her private parts into the male's nose. Through some sophisticated higher reasoning, males are able to deduce that this means the females want sex.

Estrus sex often leads to pregnancy.

We are the only mammals who don't go into estrus. Human females are unique in that they have concealed ovulation and are sexually receptive during their whole cycle. Instead of throwing themselves into nymphomania for the few days when they are ready to conceive like most mammals, *Homo sapiens* females are generally but less desperately aroused all the time. Males in our species can't tell whether a female is ready for impregnation, so no genes for the ancient male attraction to estrus survived. The vast majority of human males are not attracted to an inside-out pink butt. Instead, hominid males were under selection pressure to be attracted all month long, and to keep having sex all month long in hope of hitting the jackpot. Sex without estrus almost never leads to pregnancy.

Most human sexual intercourse serves not to impregnate but to bond. Evolutionary biologists say female *Homo sapiens* evolved sexual mystery to keep males enticed and more liable to form lasting attachments.

This dynamic coded into our bodies is also coded into our brains, causing the legendary coyness of women and cluelessness of men. Men try to figure out how to have sex with women, and women try to keep men trying to figure them out.

Secrecy causes paranoia. Take a look at how most *Homo sapiens* cultures have treated the menstrual cycle. Males run in terror and write strict rules. Females hide their menstrual cycle like it's shameful and shroud it in mysterious rituals.

No such pathology among baboons. The baboon female turns her menstrual cycle into a public pronouncement. Each day, she makes sure everyone in the group knows exactly where she is and how she feels about it. Her butt turns pink during ovulation, turns scarlet after conception, and disappears altogether when she is not fertile. Just in case there are any blind baboons in the band, each stage has its stench. Male baboons don't need to do much deep thinking to guess when to have sex with a female.

That's why baboon males are not ensnared by the mysterious reproductive possibilities of the female. They know exactly how fertile she is at any moment, set their schedules around it. Any sign of PMS, they get back to competing in the good ol' boys network. That's why baboons don't do much dad-care. Nor have they evolved the slightest sensitivity to female feelings. They don't have to. All they need to know is right there in the fragrant psychedelic booty.

Without pink butts, how are we *Homo sapiens* males supposed to know what's going on in there? So far *Homo sapiens* males have not evolved skills for reading reproductive viability in the mood swings. Even though *Homo sapiens* females have evolved the ability to synchronize their cycles with every other female in the tribe to hit males over the head with one great hormonal tidal wave, it's still too subtle for males. Can you blame us? Seven million years ago, it was all pink butts.

Male confusion doesn't end there. Soon we will find out how female apes trick males into thinking they're in charge. They're so good at it, in fact, they even fooled the male *Homo sapiens* studying them.

But first we need to find out why you're such a pervert.

13.

Why You're So Horny

Just think of the runaway process our ancestors got themselves into. Year-round sexual receptivity was favored in hominid females, which in turn selected for males to be year-round horny, which put more pressure on secretly-ovulating females to evolve further horniness, which in turn caused a runaway feedback loop in our sexual selection, causing most of the problems and delights in the ape species *Homo perverto*.

Since most hominid sex served more to bond than procreate, sexuality became more emphasized than sex. For most apes, there is little difference between flirtation and foreplay. Other apes flirt to fornicate. According to my tally of my pick-up attempts, 999/1000ths of human flirtation does not end in fornication.

A chimp scientist studying our behavior would say, "All this wasteful teasing! What's the point?"

A closer inspection of our bodies would reveal a giant, naked ape composed entirely of superfluous erogenous zones. Dangling earlobes, inside-out lips, impractically large breasts, giant penises, infantile hairless skin.

"Hmm," the chimp scientist would say.

Skin with fur likes to be scratched. Skin without fur likes to be caressed. Naked skin on apes is generally reserved for the genitals. Not so for *Homo perverto*. Our skin stays hairless and baby-like all through our breeding years. We have sexual nerves going to extraneous hot spots all over our bodies, like our inner thighs, the backs of our knees, our toes, our nipples, our necks. This is all located a long way from our genitals. A *Homo sapiens*, really, is built to be one giant genital. When you see a naked woman, you're basically seeing a giant clitoris. Men are dicks, but in a good way.

The chimp scientist would say, "All this extra sex tissue! What's the point?"

When a male chimp wants sex, he exposes the only hairless part of his body. He flicks it with his finger to display boingitude. If his inamorata exposes the only hairless part of her body, they begin boinking. They usually skip the kiss.

When a male *Homo sapiens* wants sex, his work is much more complicated. Proudly exposing his erection from a distance of 10 feet just doesn't work on a *Homo sapiens* female. Nor does leaping straight for her labia. The male *Homo sapiens* usually has to start as far away from her genitals as possible. Luckily, all roads lead to the clitoris, since almost every part of a *Homo sapiens* female's skin is an extension of her clitoris. The road from her neck to her vagina can take weeks. (Months at my college.) During our long, drawn-out process of depositing a little genetic material, a whole lot of valuable calories get burned.

The chimp scientist would say, "All this extra courtship! What's the point?"

Most of our everyday behavior is also completely superfluous. We have an urge to adorn the body, paint pictures, sings songs, build towers—none of this directly helps rear babies, aids gathering, or facilitates the hunt. All our courtship certainly doesn't conserve energy. No animal strokes, talks, smiles, flirts, and engages in as elaborate a variety of fashion and fetishism as *Homo sapiens* does. A close second is the bonobo, an ape who almost approaches the variety, but beats us in the frequency, and who, along with the chimp, is the animal most genetically similar to us.

But even bonobos aren't romantic. When's the last time you saw a male bonobo playing guitar beneath a female's tree? Other apes haven't evolved art. They don't idealize their lust interest. They have no modesty. They don't encumber their sex with all this clothing and operatic preliminaries. They just get the job done.

Baboons mate for eight seconds. Gorillas and chimps take about fifteen seconds to copulate. When you add up all the fore-play, fornication, and climax, human sex lasts on average a hundred times longer than that of most monkeys or apes. And the human scientists who made this calculation didn't even include the court-ing or post-coital cuddling. (Note to self: Insight into scientists' celibacy somewhere in here.)

It's not your fault you're a pervert. You have a pervert's brain. In the primary sensory and motor cortices in our brains, an awful lot of space is devoted to lips, tongue, genitals, and hands. And this in a brain that already has a lot of competition for space. These large areas for extra-sensitive touch evolved because foreplay became more important than philosophy. The only thing we like better than curiosity is being touched and touching. Sure I like science, but I'll take fornication over fascination any day.

At least three-quarters of fertile female *Homo sapiens* sex occurs with *zero* chance of conception, and the other quarter with a relatively slim chance compared to sex with females who go into estrus. Females of our species are unique in their desire to mate while pregnant, after menopause, and into old age.

"All this extra sex! All these extra erogenous zones! All this extra courtship! All this prime brain real estate devoted to foreplay! What is the point?"

To preserve the family. Our oversized penises and breasts and myriad perversions evolved to ensure that males baby-sit. The primary function of baboon sex is to make children. The primary function of human sex is to raise children. The human pair-bond was so important to childhood development, genes to increase omni-sexuality out-evolved genes for preserving energy for the next famine. The point of human sex is to *make* love.

Why evolve all this elaborate sexuality instead of just evolving the desire to be committed parents? Because of that persistent tension between the reproductive interests of sperm-spreaders and egg protectors. In our species, tension equals sex.

Today we complain that the public obsession with sex threatens children. But children were the ones who created the adult obsession with sex. For adults' bad morals, I blame the children.

When religious fundamentalists condemn sexual practices they consider "unnatural," they've got it all wrong. The purpose of human perversion is not procreation. The purpose of human perversion is to preserve marriage. The best way to save the family is to celebrate creative sexuality.

Isn't there more to life than sex? I spend a very small proportion of each day orgasming. Why do I put so much effort into it? Aren't there other things to do? Why is everybody obsessed with sex?

You have trillions of ancestors. Can you think of one true thing you can say about every single one of them? You can't say they were all the fittest survivors, because many died young. You can't even say they all loved, or had thoughts, or cell walls, or nuclei. You can't even say they were aware they existed.

The one true thing you can say about every single one of your trillions of ancestors is that they each reproduced. Those that didn't have offspring didn't get to be ancestors. In the race to reproduce, only the best reproducers won, every generation. Think of that. The most powerful force in our bodies and brains is the accumulated desire of all our ancestors, refined, concentrated, and made more powerful than any desire we imagine more important. With such a horny force animating every microscopic detail of our cells, we should think of all human needs as sub-needs arising from the desire to procreate. Our hunger for love, our ambitions, our desire to belong, our urge to make beautiful things, our need to talk, our voracious curiosity, our fear of death, our longing for transcendence, our willingness to die for our community, our ache for God. All our qualities evolved to the extent they served the reproduction of genes in ourselves and our beloved annoying relatives.

So if everybody is so horny, why can't you find a date? Never fear, Biology Boy will explain.

14.

Darwinism: Survival of the Sexiest

Ladies, which would you rather do: run from Los Angeles to Denver or go through a pregnancy? Both consume about 80,000 calories. When a woman risks intercourse, she risks having to run from Los Angeles to Denver, at which point her labors are only just beginning.

Fellahs, which would you rather do, watch an entire football game from your couch, or have sex with a woman? Calorie-wise, it's a toss up. If you want to satisfy the woman, too, add the pre-game show. What both activities have in common is that when they're done, they're done.

Tell me if this sounds like a good deal: a woman runs from Los Angeles to Denver, then jumps on the back of some guy, who then has to piggyback her around the planet during the breastfeeding years, which last two to four years among foraging peoples bereft of breast pumps. For the next fifteen years, the man and woman must run side-by-side around the Earth until they've burned ten to thirteen million extra calories. By the way, no resting. You stop for a rest, the kid starves. And you men don't want that to happen, because you're *pretty sure* the kid is yours. Sound good? Can women and men agree to this deal?

Why won't she sleep with you? Why can't he commit?

Women are reluctant to run from Los Angeles to Denver. Men are reluctant to piggyback a pregnant woman around the planet.

Hot women. From puberty to marriage, they're never alone. Boyfriends segue. Trying to date a hot woman is like trying to find parking in San Francisco. There's no such thing as a space that isn't taken. You wander around until one opens up right in front of you. In my city, you don't choose parking. Parking chooses you. And you gotta pay for every minute.

Take a look at the market. A whole teaspoon of one-hundred million sperm is worth fifty bucks. You need 20,000 sperm to earn one penny. One single egg fetches $50,000 on the open market, and that's not even including the womb rental, which sends prices into the stratosphere.

In capitalism, the market decides, and the market has spoken: Women are not worried about sperm shortages. They're worried about dependable piggybackers. It's the men who are worried about the limited number of eggs in the world.

If your womb was made of solid gold, it would be cheaper than the womb you actually have. No wonder women jack up the price when it comes to romantic relationships. For a lifetime of steady sex, men have to promise away a lifetime of love and labor. On the Pleistocene savanna, there was no other way to raise help-less blobs of flesh to be sarcastic teenagers.

For a woman, looking for an eligible man is like playing *Where's Waldo?* Anybody with a womb had better be a smart shopper. Anybody who makes worthless sperm had better find a unique way to distinguish himself from the crowd, and the best way to do that is to display nesting potential.

When I graduated from college as an English major, my parents nagged me about getting a job and making a buck. But I was above all that. Was a man's worth measured by his dollar amount? Could the infinite potentialities of my character be reduced to mere economic worth? Bah! I was going to be a poet!

So far, none of my poems has gotten me any dates. I had some profound private moments, sure, and some women even professed appreciation for my metaphors. (Or were they similes? I can never remember the difference.) Poems get the verbal vote. But between poems and paychecks, women have voted with their vaginas.

A man wears a tie not just because it's a giant arrow that points to his crotch. It's also a symbol of success. The paycheck represents the nest. The poem represents the promise.

Never forget the evolutionary power of female choice to mold sperm-makers. Remember the principle of the peacock's tail. If females have some power of mate choice, female tastes will emerge in male bodies and behavior in a few generations.

The Watusi tribe from Rwanda and Burundi conduct something like a Miss America pageant, except the men are the contestants and the women are the judges. In a fantastic courtship ritual that has to be seen to be believed, eligible bachelors leap and dance before the single women, then await their choices. Watusi women prefer tall statures, clear eyes, long noses, healthy teeth and, most importantly, the highest jumpers. As a result of female tastes, males of this tribe have evolved bulging white eyes, great white teeth, long equine noses, extreme height, and thinness. Some are eight feet tall. They all look like Manute Bol, the 7'7" basketball player who hails from the Dinka tribe from this region. And these guys can high-jump like nobody's business. If the Watusi enter the Olympics, we're in big trouble.

The Watusi are in East Central Africa. In West Central Africa, pygmies on the singles scene don't care much about height. A few generations back, males and females decided the perfect measure of health is healthy buttocks. This caused what biologists call "steatopygia," otherwise known as a fat ass. If you're short and suffer from steatopygia, visit a pygmy village and you'll be a big hit.

The average height of the Watusi in Rwanda is 6'5". The Mbuti pygmies in the Congo average 4'4". The world's tallest and world's shortest people live a few hundred miles from each other, and it's all because of gals' fashions in guys. Our turn-ons build our bodies and brains.

Any male peacock has the genes to produce an efflorescent tail, but only those peacocks with the power to acquire lots of nutrition can. The peacock's tail is like an American's big house, a Watusi's big body, a pygmy's big butt. It is a display of conspicuous consumption. It announces, "See how powerful I am among peacocks! Let's get it on!"

This gives females goddess-like power over how males get built. We are the first species to learn we have this power. Among Pleistocene australopithecines, *ergasters*, *erectuses*, *habilines*, and archaic *Homo sapiens*, women's choice became human salvation.

15.

How Kindness Became Sexy

The first ape to talk probably brokered a deal. Our survival as hunting and gathering apes competing with lions and tigers relied crucially on debts paid and repaid over time. The best thing anybody could do to rear more babies to adulthood was to secure connections in the community. Responsible citizenship became "a visible sign of reproductive fitness." This is a biologist's technical term for the quality that makes yo' sexy ass all that. It means mates can *choose* for this trait. As hominids got better at detecting trickery, genes for fake altruism didn't survive as well as genes for sincere altruism. Hominid males, for instance, become unique in their real desire to care for youngsters and elders of their tribe. Then along comes a discriminating female.

Females can randomly evolve genes for being attracted to any quality they want—long tails, asymmetrical claws, giant penises, mental retardation, bower building—but only those qualities that lead to more surviving babies will pay off. Females who happen to be attracted to the right qualities will pass on more genes than females who are attracted to qualities that make offspring less likely to survive. A hominid gene for attraction to stupidity would be at a disadvantage compared to a gene for attraction to intelligence, whereas female black widow genes for attraction to stupidity have definitely paid off reproductively, since the replication of spider genes relies crucially on dopey dad getting eaten during sex.

Ladies, don't beat yourself up for that last moron you dated. I'm sure the female black widow is kicking herself with all eight legs for some of the smart spiders she's dated. She's a female; we all know what she really wants: to settle down with a sexy, stupid, savory spider, which couldn't provide for babies if it killed him—so she will.

A female or male shark that chose mates based on altruism and a talent for metaphors would be choosing genes that would hurt their offspring's chances for survival, because shark survival does not depend crucially on altruism and a talent for metaphors. Since the great reproductive virtues of hominids were *cooperation* and *communication*, hominids that chose mates for altruism and metaphor facility made more surviving babies than hominids that chose mates based on dorsal fins or how tasty their brains were during sex.

Our ancestors hit the evolutionary jackpot when their "primary fitness indicator"—biologese for *mojo*—became not their muscles, speed, brow ridges, or ferocity, but their minds. Other species chose mates based on criteria like tail colors, odor, succulence, or dance display. What got us mated was what we had to say. Since we need cooperation for procreation, our primary fitness indicator became how responsibly we behaved.

Whatever body part shrinks fast in evolution shrinks because it stops getting you sex. Whatever body part grows fast in evolution grows because it gets you more sex.

If a body part changes slowly or stays stable over evolutionary time, all it's doing is keeping you alive.

Right about the time *habilis* transitioned into *erectus* two million years ago, you started to see big canine teeth on males getting smaller, and male-female size ratios getting less pronounced. This means males toned down the physical fighting, and females stopped sleeping around so much and raised their standards of choosing. At the same time, you started to see brains getting bigger in both males and females. This means males and females started mentally competing more—through charm, gossip, poetry, smack-talking. As friendship and fathering skills started raising more surviving babies than fighting and fornicating skills, female choice mattered more. What got you mated wasn't who you beat up any more, so much as how clever you were, how many friends you had, what kind of parent you might make. We had to bullshit our way into each other's beds.

Sure, for a while, female hominids probably swooned for male fangs. But as social skills started rearing more surviving babies than fangs, any female turned on by scintillating conversations passed on more genes than females turned on by dopes with fangs. Soon fangs became a liability, since they use up calcium for no reason. Sure, you can bite your egghead rival, but if fangs don't get you chicks, what's their point? Maybe fangs of ferocity competed directly with words of wit, and hominids that settled disputes with bite instead of brain were thought crude, coarse—even primitive.

Maybe bullies got excluded from all the stag-eating parties. Cleverness and kindness became the real turn-ons.

Barbara Smuts of the University of Michigan, Ann Arbor has shown that over-aggressive baboon males are shunned by females for males who are more socially graceful. Maybe after a million years of males competing for female choice, baboon males will be holding doors open for their beloved babettes.

Men and women have radically different breasts, butts, hair tufts, shoulders, and waists, because hominid men and women were attracted to different physical qualities in each other.

But the similarity in men and women's cognitive abilities means that—once intelligence surpassed physicality as our primary fitness indicator—hominid males and females found empathy and intelligence equally attractive in each other. This started a runaway process. You can't judge intelligence unless you yourself are intelligent. As hominids got better at detecting trickery, genes for faking generosity would not do as well as genes for sincere generosity. Hominids mated their way to big brains and big hearts.

Add 100,000 generations to this breeding tournament, you end up with a species like us: friendly, creative, talkative, ready to outwit our rivals, manipulative, unconscious of our motives, and sincerely nice. Men and women bred each other for these qualities. Sex saved us, made us the great species we are today.

Ten thousand people in thirty-seven cultures were asked to rank thirteen qualities in a potential mate. Many sex differences were consistent across all cultures and confirmed what was predicted by evolutionary theory. But there was one way that both sexes were identical. "Kindness" was rated in the top three out of thirteen qualities by both genders in all cultures. In fact, in thirty-two of the thirty-seven cultures, men and women gave "kindness" the exact same ranking.

All our most humane qualities we owe to the opposite sex. Anything you don't like about the other gender came about by the choices of your gender. Look at the nearest members of the opposite sex. Your sex created them, body and soul. For your talents, you have to thank them and all the sex they gave you. When Hamlet waxed philosophical about our species: "how noble in reason, how infinite in faculties . . . in action how like an angel, in apprehension how like a god" [Act II, scene 2, lines 327-330], he never imagined that human beings were created by four-foot-high apes, making choices about what they thought was best in a parent and lover. Make sure you keep having sex with smart, compassionate *Homo sapiens*. It's your duty to the species.

16.

Why We Bitch

I know your psychotherapist's greatest fantasy. Just once, she would love to say, "Bitch, bitch, bitch. Is that all you ever do?"

Shut up about your mother already. There was nothing she could do about you. She can't help it if you're a *Homo sapien*.

Everybody is negative because human beings are problem solvers. Our brains are predisposed to focus on what isn't working and obsess about it.

After all, there are lots of things that go right in our civilization. So far I haven't experienced a famine, nor have marauders come to rape my daughter or take my stuff. That running water thing is a plus as well. I wrote this on a computer, it got published and printed, and now you're reading it in the future. My clock radio woke me up from my ergonomic pillow and predicted the weather for me. I woke up almost blind, but my sight was magically restored by these cheap plastic thingies that adhere to my eyeballs. Hundreds of humans put thousands of man-hours into all the ingredients in my breakfast, most of which got shipped from around the world: pepper, salt, salmon, eggs, broccoli, pesticides, and the iron, niacin, riboflavin and other stuff that went into my single slice of wheat bread. All the brainpower that was invested into making the machines that wove the microfibers of my sheets and clothes to perfect softness went off without a hitch. Vaccines protected me from disease, soap removed germs from my skin, a magic machine washed my dishes. Why aren't I in a cheerful mood?

Because my damn toaster does the damn bread with one side extra-toasted and the other side half-toasted, and every morning I have to face the same trauma of whether I should over-toast one side and under-toast the other side, or set the toaster on half-toast and push the button down twice, and I don't see why I should have to go out and buy a whole new toaster when any sane assessment of the situation decrees that the entire toaster industry deserves to be punished by my boycott.

Human brains are not built to appreciate. They're built to scrutinize for problems, propose solutions, complain until something gets done. If we participate in solving a problem, our glands reward us with a surge of chemical satisfaction. We recalibrate our sense of self-esteem accordingly. You can see success in someone's bearing. Then, immediately, we go to the next problem, take old successes for granted, start slouching again. Human nature is built not for satisfaction but progress. You thrive not by surviving but by striving.

The only reason I even bring this up is to bitch about it. You won't see me appreciating my toilet any time soon. I don't care how much it saved civilization from medieval diseases and butt rot.

Why aren't they self-cleaning?

I define Murphy's Law as the tendency for humans to notice what doesn't go right. Let me also define Quirk's Law: Almost everything in civilization is perpetually and simultaneously going right, and nobody will ever notice.

Look at this paragraph. I had to write these words. Somebody had to copyedit it for grammar and spelling. Somebody had to typeset it one letter at a time. The design, the printing, the binding, the marketing that finds the audience and puts the book in your hands—it all had to go right. The number of tiny details that could have been screwed up is astronomical, yet almost all of it worked out in a superhuman surge of cooperative competence that spontaneously occurs among humans whenever money (reproductive currency) is at stake. The production, copying, and distribution of this paragraph in this book was a titanic achievement, and we pulled it off.

You know what I'm upset about? The font. I wanted Antique Gothic with ten more pages. I think the weight of my subject deserves something grand and spread out. They got me Bembo with ten fewer pages. Financial considerations. But it looks all squishy. I don't see why Mr. Big-Shot Carl Sagan gets Antique Gothic when I have to settle for Bembo. I'm finding out who's responsible, and giving them hell. This whole book, in my opinion, is screwed up. Bembo, indeed.

Are any of the hundreds, nay, thousands of people involved in this process happy? Nope. We're all stressed out, angry with the other guy, keeping track of each and every foul-up that made everything a last-minute panic rush.

Teachers had to teach us how to read. Factories had to provide paper. Horses had to provide glue. Planes and trucks had to ship it to stores. Inventories had to be kept. Everybody had to be paid. Taxes had to be deducted. It all had to be added up ahead of time to make sure we all came out ahead of the red.

Does anybody sit around appreciating this stuff? No. It's too much trouble to notice all the things that go right. There's too much of it. Somehow it's just more efficient to focus on the screw-ups. If we didn't, we wouldn't be the kick-ass species that we are.

Are you grouchy today? Blame your thumb.

Other animals don't frown at the world and see a shoddy job that needs to be fixed. Once *Homo habilis* evolved an opposable thumb that could minutely use tools, there was strong competition to see the world as a series of technical problems that needed to be solved. Complaining is how a tool-user searches for problems. A perpetual sense of dissatisfaction really helps you find them. Lots of animals suffer from cold, darkness, and hunger. Only problem-solving tool-users came up with fire, the wheel, and agriculture, yet still bitch that the restaurant is drafty.

Deep in your genome is the Bitching Gene. It got selected for by millennia of tool-using apes competing to seek and solve problems. He who didn't bitch didn't solve the problems that led to babies, the biggest problems of all.

Lizards don't complain. Zebras don't complain. Fish are pretty stoic. But give birth to a human being, and what's the first thing it does? Complain. Loudly. As soon as that womb is gone, we notice something is wrong, and we call everybody's attention to it:

"We have a problem here. I have a mouth, and there is no breast in it. I have some gas. Somebody do something about that. The temperature just offended my sensibilities. Why can't we keep everything at optimum comfort levels? If somebody would predict my needs before they occur to me, we wouldn't have this problem.

Maybe I want some stimulus jiggled in front of my face, or maybe I want to be driven around in the car. I'm not sure. Keep guessing until I figure it out. Stop feeding me, I want to nap. It wouldn't kill you to rock my cradle. C'mon, people! Incompetence, incompetence, everywhere I look! I'm surrounded by idiots!"

These are the first thoughts humans have. A human infant who can scarcely focus his eyes has an amazing ability to convey indignant outrage. A toddler's hauteur seems to me unearned by his experience. My cousin's four-year-old kid issues queenly edicts I can't imagine coming from a wombat or a sea squirt.

Newborn cows, newborn seahorses, newborn turtles come into the world not expecting much. Newborn humans come into the world expecting the world. From there on out, it's one big disappointment. Everyone we meet is the complaint department. To bitch is to bond. There's little that so bonds humans like a shared annoyance.

Ever meet one of those genetic mutants who's just so damn chipper about everything? Don't you want to just slap them? You know why you want to slap them? To give them something to complain about. Then you'll have something to bond about.

Don't think I don't know that all the wonderful things I just listed about civilization didn't make you want to smack me. That's why I wrote it in a book, instead of mentioning it to my friends. I don't want them to notice my optimism problem. "Man, shut up with the appreciation already!" they'll say. "Don't you read the papers?"

What's up with the papers? They shouldn't call it news. They should call it bad news. All sorts of wonderful stuff happened yesterday: babies got born, friendships were forged, money was made, sex was had. Who wants to read about that crap in the papers? The news media is a colossal machine that scrutinizes the globe for every piece of bad news and brings it into our living rooms to satisfy our unquenchable desire to obsess about problems.

Poets express deep eternal longings. Most poems satisfy the deepest, most eternal longing of all: the yearning to whine. Thank goodness Keats lived before Prozac. I can't get enough of his melancholia. If he wasn't yearning and pining, he wouldn't speak to me so deeply. He'd just sound like Dr. Seuss. Happy art is shallow. Sad art is deep. Depressing movies, tragic novels, stark paintings, sad songs: those are profound. Uplifting movies, upbeat novels, romantic paintings, happy love songs: those are trite. For our masochistic taste in art, we can thank the Bitching Gene.

Without the Bitching Gene, we never would have conquered the Earth and ruined it for all the other large species. There would only be a few thousand of us, and nobody would have invented the alphabet. Problem-solving hominid species who sat around appreciating everything didn't put the full weight of their brain power behind obsessing about new problems, and thus didn't pass on as many genes as problem-solving species who did nothing but concentrate on problems.

When *Homo sapiens* stumbled on the Neanderthal, we were carrying a whole bunch of superior technology we had invented because of our tendency to see everything as a problem to be solved. We took one look at the muscular, bigger-brained Neanderthal and saw another problem. We promptly solved it.

That's how genes for kvetching got selected for. Once problem-solving became crucial to hominid reproductive viability, it was inevitable that the whiniest of all hominid species would outcompete all others, including the more athletic ones with bigger brains. I'm going to end this book on the inspiring truth that, genetically, all humans are one big family. But this is true only because we killed all the other families.

In fact, in any species where the increased solving of problems confers a reproductive advantage, a gene for being predisposed to see only problems would get selected for. To build an organism to be the best solution-seeker in nature, make them blind to what goes right. In fact, make that organism remember what goes right only to the extent it teaches him what to do next time. This habit is called "taking things for granted."

Look at you. Your luxurious life is about as different from your Pleistocene ancestors' as it can get. Modern civilization fulfilled every dream of Pleistocene hominids, then invented new dreams and satisfied those. Yet you still possess your Pleistocene bitching brain.

Civilizations of the past dreamed of the Land of Milk and Honey, where wine flowed in rivers and food flew into our mouths. Today we can get all the milk and honey we want. My beer keg flows until I'm stupefied, and pizzas fly to my front door.

Not so long ago, people killed, died, and traveled thousands of miles along the Silk Road for such rare delicacies as salt and pepper. They suffered and died dreaming of heaven, where these exotic luxuries would be at their fingertips.

Heaven was a place where mankind did not have to labor by the sweat of its brow. Ancient laborers envied the un-calloused hands and soft bellies of royalty. Ancient kings shipped in entertainers from all over their lands to entertain them.

Few of us sweat at work. When was the last time you had a callus? We flick through five hundred channels of free entertainment twenty-four hours a day, complaining that nothing is on.

We live in ancient paradises. The United States is the Land of Milk and Honey. You'd think paradise would satisfy us.

Hell, no. The biggest problem in modern daily life is the

absence of problems. Think about it. What is the main complaint
of middle-class Americans? The same complaint of medieval kings.
We're bored! That's why we spend so much time seeking entertainment, which is pretend conflict. "Can't we get a little drama
around here?" we ask. We forget that drama is a synonym for a
problem, the source of stress, and stimulator of the Bitching Gene.

Peasants weren't bored, people starving in Bangladesh aren't
bored, and your Pleistocene grandmother was not bored. Boredom
comes from the absence of challenges. Only a problem-seeking
species can get bored. Your mean boss, clogged traffic, your pothead
teenager, your stolen car—those aren't real problems. Saber-toothed
tigers, malnourished infants, Black Plague, armies paid to extermi-
nate you—those are the problems that built your brain. Obsessing
about them was a good idea.

Now look at us. Brains built to bellyache placed in an environment of supermarkets, cyber-sex, and central heating. It would
look like a pretty sweet deal to an australopithecine. Yet we still
look at our world through Pleistocene glasses. Everything we see is
a problem that needs to be fixed.

Gravity is a problem. We need to invent flying. Mortality
inconveniences me. No, I don't want to stop eating bacon burgers!
Somebody invent triple bypass surgery instead!

What the hell is going on at the bottom of the ocean anyway?
It is so my business! Invent something!

The fact that that star is just sitting up there, and I don't know
what it's doing, really burns me up. When is that problem going to
be solved? Put a team on that; I expect up-to-the-minute reports.

Come to think of it, I'm not satisfied with my genes.
Evolution's text needs some editing. Start the Genome Project!
Actually, I'm not satisfied with anything's genes. Tomatoes could

certainly stand an upgrade. Hop on that job, Monsanto!

Why should I have to wiggle my wrist while brushing my teeth? What am I, a slave? Put an electric motor in my toothbrush!

Bitch, bitch, bitch. Our ancestors had to organize big groups to out-hunt man-eating lions, out-gather giant herbivores and insects, drag a giant boar home, cook it, and eat it without anybody raiding them for it. It was a full-day chore.

Now we pull frozen dinners out of the freezer, then tap our foot complaining that the microwave takes five whole minutes to cook it! Don't kid yourself that fulfilling one more desire will satisfy our species.

If we can't find any problems, we'll make them up. Archaeologists found evidence that red ochre make-up and probably deodorant were used 110,000 years ago. Asian *Homo erectus* didn't worry that the natural scent of his own self needed to be masked with a fake scent. He was too busy running from us. We deodorant-wearing apes were his biggest problem. He never solved us. We solved him.

Solving problems requires a tremendous amount of food energy. Smart primates spend 8% of their calories on their brains. We spend 20% to 25% of our calories on our brains, and our brains are only 2% of our body weight.

That's why we obsess more than we scamper. Take your dog to the park, and you'll know what I mean. Dog: scampering. You: obsessing about problems, including the problem of why you can't be more carefree, like your dog.

Look at him. Just scampering away and sniffing butts as if life is something to be enjoyed. The moron. Doesn't he see all the problems?

Because of the evolutionary accident of our thumbs, the

tremendous food energy spent on solving problems paid off reproductively for us. The tremendous food energy spent on scampering
and butt-sniffing paid off for the dog, probably in hunting and
social skills. Human natural selection sacrificed scampering for
brain power. Studies in butt-sniffing are yet to be funded, but you
can bet that the amount of food energy we spend on compulsive
scampering and sniffing is equivalent to the amount of food energy
my dog spends on his brain.

All adaptations work within this energy-for-reproductive-viability trade-off. Hummingbirds gave it all to the extraordinary ability
to hover like a helicopter, but this energy cost is so high, the hummingbird had to sacrifice size, and she has to eat a meal a minute,
all day, every day, then go into a hibernation when she sleeps that
looks more like death than coma.

For every trait in an organism, there is a cost/benefit tradeoff.
Genes blindly create qualities. So long as the reproductive benefit
of any quality outweighs the cost, the quality will increase.

The tremendous cost of a peacock's tail—in energy, in foliage
entanglements, in its free-meal advertisement to predators—has so
far been outweighed by the tremendous sexual benefits of its ability
to woo peahens. Until the reproductive cost of the tail outweighs the
reproductive benefit of the tail, the tail will keep getting bigger. In
other words, so long as the tail gets him more sex than death, peacock tails will grow.

This is true with any organism's trait. Our ability to seek and
solve problems conferred a reproductive benefit that outweighed
its cost in energy. Our brains are calibrated to be precisely as smart
as paid off reproductively in our ancestral environment. It remains
to be seen if our ability to out-think ourselves will pay off reproductively in the next million years. There's no reason why genes

won't select for *Homo sapiens* to become stupider, a Homo slightly less sapient. I'm not sure a little less brain power and little more scampering would be a bad thing. Maybe we'll evolve into *Homo scampus sniffus*.

Until then, keep complaining. Remember that the noble search for problems and solutions is what caused us to always see the negative side of everything. We owe all our good stuff to our inability to appreciate it. For that we should be grateful.

17.

Why We Are Fat

Don't beat yourself up. It's a primate problem.

The athletic orangutan, swinging from tree to tree looking for food, weighs in at a lean 160 pounds. The male orangutan is so content to be alone for weeks, primatologists have described him as Zen–like, the very embodiment of dignity.

Then there's Pumpkin. (The name has been changed to protect the subject from embarrassment.) Pumpkin lived in the Atlanta zoo and was the life of the party. Painted lovely pictures. Learned 150 sign-language words. Charmed every child he met. A real showman. Playful as a pup.

A big fat pup. Pumpkin weighed 500 pounds. Wild orangutans wouldn't even recognize the corpulent Pumpkin. He ate so much; primatologists became concerned that his blubber would collapse his lungs. They put him on a diet.

Now, Pumpkin was not only fat but mean. Remember your last diet? Now imagine if that diet was enforced, and you had no vanity and no sense of propriety. Pumpkin refused to paint, ate his Crayons, wouldn't sign except in reference to food, tossed some feces. Pumpkin was no longer the chief attraction at the zoo.

Finally, Pumpkin staged a breakout. The zookeepers panicked. A hungry, grouchy, well-trained orangutan on the loose! Pumpkin could easily kill a man, climb any structure. They wouldn't put it past Pumpkin to try to operate a vehicle. They checked the closets, the local woods, and the roof. "Think like an orangutan!" the zookeepers shouted to each other. "Where would you go if you were an obese orangutan on a diet?"

Pumpkin was found in the kitchen, using all four hands to stuff the entire contents of a fifty-five-gallon drum of monkey chow into his face.

Pumpkin had to be sedated and restrained. Hosed off. Dragged kicking and roaring back to his playland habitat, his folds of orange flab squeaking across the tile floor. It was not a day of Zen-like dignity for Pumpkin.

Why did I just put you through that horror story? To illustrate a concept in evolutionary biology. In nature, there are two feeding strategies: animals are either hoarders or gorgers. It all depends on whether you eat perishable food.

Put yourself on the savanna. You just killed the last short-necked giraffid in Africa with your Pleistocene buddies. You're throwing rocks at the salivating hyenas. Your mate is waiting at home with a big basket of berries. The Ice Age is not only a few millennia off, it's thousands of miles away, so don't even think about refrigeration. Here come the flies.

When food goes rancid fast, and food comes infrequently and in huge amounts, your best bet is to stuff your face, Pumpkin-style. The next famine is always a week away. The overriding purpose of eating is to store fat. Most mammals are built to eat all they can get. But what happens if you can get all you want?

Obesity was invented by civilization. We Americans are fat because we're so darn efficient at storing food energy. Cut off our food supply, it takes us two months to die, three months for the super-plump. Now that's storing.

If you were a squirrel, you'd hoard. Nuts last. Why store your energy on your butt when you can store it in a tree? When winter hits, squirrels recover more than 80% of their thousands of buried nuts. Famine, shmamine. Squirrels know how to invest. Trim, sleek, athletic, diligent, squirrels are an evolutionary biologist's classic example of a hoarder.

How I admire them. Once, when I shot, skinned, cooked, and devoured one, I was amazed at how dense and muscular the cute little guy was. Not one gram of fat on him.

I was pretty full after two squirrels. I ate three.

But even if you're nature's patron saint of frugality, civilization has a way of corrupting even animals genetically programmed for temperance.

The Grand Canyon. Ancient as Earth. Cathedral of the Titans. And home of the Kamikaze squirrel.

Every time I stopped for a snack, I was surrounded. Roving gangs of obese, double-chinned, salivating squirrels were everywhere. They don't beg. They snap at your McNugget while you're trying to eat it. They dive into your backpack while you're wearing it. I don't think anybody has obeyed the "DON'T FEED THE WILDLIFE" signs in the history of tourism. After generations of living off Twinkies and Snack-Packs, these squirrels wouldn't know a nut if you threw it at them, and I threw quite a few. Ripping into my trail mix, they ignored the nuts and went after the M&M's. Watching one from behind, waddling off with my French fry, was less than charming. There's nothing more depressing than being mugged by a fat squirrel.

My friends and I were the only humans down in the rugged section of the Grand Canyon who weren't speaking German and eating astronaut food out of tubes. We were also the only humans who were portly, gasping, and stopping every half-mile to consume our Happy Meals. I couldn't help wondering if these striding uber-hikers noticed that even the squirrels seemed American.

We are fat because gorgers are biologically designed to eat more than they need. Put a gorger in an environment where food supply is infinite and requires no exercise to get, he's going to be fat. Our unnatural diet can even seduce the Grand Canyon squirrel, an animal genetically programmed for hoarding!

Next time you feel guilty about your binge, remember Pumpkin. Eating that entire bag of Doritos doesn't seem so self-indulgent when you think of Pumpkin and his fifty-five-gallon drum.

But before we break into the Ding Dongs in despair, look at your rolling folds and thank them for the evolution of humanity. As we'll see in the next chapter, our brains might never have gotten so big without our fat asses. All our extra blubber came in handy when it was time to float.

18.

Aqua-Ape: The Missing Link?

Throw a chimp into a lake, he's dead. Apes can't swim, float, or hold their breath. Where did we learn to swim, float, and hold our breath?

Early hominid settlements are almost always found alongside water. Most of our cities have since been built next to water. Why is waterfront property so valuable? What's the point of lying half-naked on a beach doing nothing? Why all the boating, snorkeling, water polo, and squirt gun fights? Why install swimming pools in our backyards?

There's a big gap in the fossil record between the time we were tree-swinging fruit-eaters and the time we were sprinting around on the savanna cutting down big game. What was going on in that 1.5 million-year interim between *Orrorin tugenesis* and *Ardipithecus ramidus*, and why can't we find one measly fossil? Seems mighty fishy.

We and chimps split from our common ancestor roughly six million years ago. At that time, Africa, where we lived, was experiencing great rises and falls of sea level. Climates changed and threatened food supplies. Our apish ancestors were getting pushed out of the jungle competition for food. Suppose our ancestral grandmother saw seaweed glistening temptingly in the waves, or fish darting in the swamps beneath her tree.

Chimpy tries a little wading, just like we see modern macaques doing. She eats more than her friends. Genes for water facility begin to be favored. Bipedal wading starts to evolve. Soon there is swimming and diving. A niche is colonized.

The Aquatic Ape hypothesis is getting some strong backing among experts. Other experts say the Aqua-Ape theory is all wet. Here's the evidence. You decide if it sinks or swims.

We're one weird-looking ape. We're naked. Most other naked mammals are the ones who returned to the waters. We have streamlined bodies, which are perfect for swimming. We are the only apes that have hair on our backs that curls backward and inward toward our spine, which aids water flow.

Next time you see a gorilla, dump a bucket of water on him. Make sure you are on the other side of the bars. Not only will it piss him off, you will see his hair actually resist the flow of the water. Now watch your arm hairs in the shower. Doesn't piss you off at all, does it? We love to bathe, and our bodies are elegantly hydrodynamic.

Of course, we're not completely hairless. There is a prominent tuft of hair on the top of our heads.

Ever see a bunch of kids playing in a pool? We don't stay under for as long as dolphins and whales. Most of the time, human heads are above water. We might have retained the hair on top of our heads while we were dog paddling around. It prevented sunstroke. Heat travels up and exits out the top of our heads, and hair cuts down on that considerably. Note how often kids play games of diving to find objects at the bottom.

Walking ape-like with knuckles and short legs is good. Walking upright with long legs is good. But walking in the stooped in-between stage is terribly awkward and inefficient. We needed a million years or so to transition from knuckle-draggers to we of noble stature. For this stooped locomotion to have worked for so long, it must have accorded us tremendous benefits to offset the tremendous disadvantage of being a waddling hunter ape. Maybe a million years of wading into deeper waters for more delectable seafood slowly stood us upright to keep our head above water, until we learned to dive and swim. In *The Life of Mammals*, David Attenborough shows amazing footage of chimps standing upright to wade across open water.

Perhaps we developed tool-use to break open mollusks.

And what's with all our subcutaneous fat? Other apes store their fat like a terrestrial animal should, shoved down between their kidneys and intestines. All over our bodies, just under our skin, we spread a plush pillow top of pudge—just like all aquatic mammals.

Fat is buoyant, an excellent insulator in water. Even the thinnest of us has ten times as many fat cells as other land animals our size.

Try teaching a gorilla how to swim. He'll never get it. Yet humans are born knowing how to swim. Human babies are expert floaters and instinctively hold their breaths when they go under. It's healthy for human mothers to give birth in water.

Humans don't learn how to swim. We forget how to swim. The rolls of billowing baby fat we find so cute might be for babies dropped from trees into water.

Think I'm joking? Brave parents can literally hurl their new-borns into a pool. The babies splash into the water, instinctively hold their breath until they surface, then back float smiling and breathing and kicking their feet with nary a tear.

And tears. Ever see an orangutan cry? The only mammals that produce salty tears of emotion are marine mammals and us. Seals and sea otters weep tears when they've lost their young. We're the only land animal that has this aquatic trait.

For runners on the hot savanna, we sure sweat and pee a lot. This is a shameful waste of water. Other land animals in Africa drink and urinate much less. It's as if we think we're in an environment where we can get all the water we want. Our sweat is also oily, of a kind used by aquatic mammals to waterproof their hair follicles.

We speak. We can do this in part because we can choose to hold our breath. Other primates can't talk, because they can't hold their breath, and they can't breathe well through their mouths. They also can't choke to death on a bone, as we can. Using the same tube to eat and breathe is a dangerous adaptation, especially when you have a perfectly good nose to breathe through—even more especially when toddlers want to put every throat-sized object in their mouths. Why would we evolve to hold our breath?

Let's check the list of animals that have voluntary breath control: seals, dolphins, and us.

To aid our breath control, we have a "descended" larynx. What other animals have this feature? The sea-lion, walrus, and manatee.

Mouth breathing also allows you to take in a very deep breath—before a dive, for instance. We even have a nose shaped like a half-pyramid, which protects our nostrils from a dive. If a gorilla falls head-first into a pool, his straight-out nostrils allow his sinuses to fill with water, and he immediately drowns.

Marine mammals have a "diving reflex." When an otter's face hits water, specialized nerves in his mouth and nose shut off the passage to his lungs, slow his heart rate, and send blood directly to his vital organs. Humans have this diving reflex. Other primates do not. Immersion in water up to our necks actually soothes us, while it causes panic in most mammals.

We have big brains, even bigger than other primates. Who else has brains that big? Dolphins. Whales, too. Is there something about an aquatic environment that selects for big brains? Absolutely. The building of massive brain tissue depends upon the Omega-3 fatty acids found most abundantly in fish.

We are also unique among apes in that Omega 3 fish fats are actually good for us. Where would we have found fish on the dry savanna? We savanna hunters have health problems with animal fat and vegetable fat, yet we evolved to utilize fish fats with optimum efficiency. Did we start eating fish in preference to wildebeest?

Take a look at your teeth. For an African hunter, you have lame fangs compared to a baboon. The teeth of early australopithecine, our direct ancestor, more closely resemble those of the sea otter. Rough plant fiber and raw animal flesh was better masticated by our cousin the Neanderthal. Our teeth are better suited to softer flesh and to cracking open sea shells. Land animal meat we prefer to soften up with a little cooking, which is a form a pre-digestion. Tigers don't need burnt meat. They can digest it raw. Then again, they can't digest raw sushi or chew seaweed.

Look at the space between the thumb and forefinger of a monkey or an ape, and there seems to be something missing. The slight webbing between our fingers and toes might be vestigial. You may be shocked to know that 7% of humans have webbed toes.

In fact, most of the traits we possess that are different from chimps' are traits we share with marine mammals.

The transition from a water-hating primate to a water-loving primate is easy to make. It's so easy, in fact, scientists witnessed it in one generation. The Japanese Macaques of the Koshima Islet picked scattered grain out of the beach sand, yet never went into the waves. A two-year-old macaque discovered that if he threw handfuls of sand into the ocean, the sand sunk and the grain floated to the top. He scooped up the floating grain and ate faster than anyone. When his young peers saw this, they imitated his innovation, and soon these young rebels were splashing and playing in the waves for the first time. The elders disapproved. The old farts ate less grain than the youngsters. They got old and died, taking their stodgy old culture with them. A new generation of macaques came of age, and body-surfing has since become a permanent feature of the island species' behavior.

Do our religious baptisms play out our primeval baptism? Our poetry often is about returning to the water. I don't think the poet's muse is referring all the way back to when we were fish climbing up on land to lay eggs. Nobody wants to get in touch with his inner fish.

Why should every culture have a Flood Myth anyway? Maybe our dreams of flying are actually dreams of swimming! Hey, come to think of it, our superheroes fly with streamlined bodies! Our gods float weightlessly! Maybe our myths of mermaids are actually our genetic memories of when we were mer-apes!

And this is where the Aquatic Ape theory gets into trouble. The speculation is endless. Once you grab onto a hypothesis, you find more and more arguments to support it. It becomes like the Kennedy assassination.

The only thing the Aquatic Ape hypothesis has going for it is tremendous explanatory power. It doesn't have even one piece of hard scientific evidence, such as a bone, or the fossilized imprint of a webbed hominid foot that's more specialized for swimming than just a couple webbed toes.

Aquatic Ape enthusiasts say it's not their fault there's no evidence. Glaciers encroached and receded during the Pleistocene, creating great changes in sea level. The rich coastlines and shallow seas which Pleistocene hominids must have exploited are now covered by deep ocean which has obliterated archaeological evidence. We don't know what these coastline hominids looked like, but many believe they used boats.

Aquatic ape enthusiasts are calling for anthropologists to search for fossils under the waves in hopes that they might find the legendary "missing link." They say the Aquatic Ape hypothesis is the only theory that explains bipedalism, conscious breath control, reduced body hair, and subcutaneous fat.

Other experts have offered an alternative theory. They propose that maybe we haven't found any amphibious ape bones because— duh!—there's no such thing as an aquatic ape!

What's that? How will this help you get loved and laid?

Well, excuse *me* for a fascinating diversion into scientific theory! Fine, back to the sex! Sheesh.

My training as an amateur anthropologist should have given me power to predict that you would prefer to hear more about sex. Pleistocene dynamics created everything we viscerally react to. Which do you like more? Shakespeare or Spielberg? As an amateur ethologist trained to observe behavior, I am not interested in what you say you like. I am interested in what you choose to experience.

19.

Why You Like Spielberg More than T. S. Eliot

Evolutionary biology has all the elements of a soap opera: Love and sex! Violence and compassion! Teamwork and conspiracies! Marriage and infidelity! Child-rearing and chases! Loyalty and betrayal! And family, family, family! We can even throw in a slap-fight between adulteresses. No matter how hard the science dweebs try to make this stuff boring, this burgeoning field of research is destined for the front pages of *Maxim*, *Cosmopolitan*, and *Seventeen*. We've got to get it right before Jerry Springer gets his hands on it.

The reason we react instinctively to soap operas is that they play out ancient dramas. The reason we find it a guilty pleasure is that our neocortexes tell us the soap opera writers are cynically pushing all the Pleistocene buttons that get us going. You can

WHY YOU LIKE SPIELBERG MORE THAN T. S. ELIOT   111

almost hear them proposing the next script:

"Have Rebecca sleep with Lance who's married to her sister Destiny with whom she is in competition for the inheritance, then have Destiny walk in on them, then end the episode as the sisters make eye contact. We'll pick up on that storyline five episodes later. Right now we have to get back to Alexandra falling in love with her kidnapper."

Subtlety, shmubtlety. This crap is automatically dramatic. I believe it was Aristotle, in his treatise on poetics, who first declared, "The stupid is always dramatic."

Well, I'm paraphrasing, but you know what I mean.

Blame the brain. Or rather, blame all three of your brains. Why can't they just get along?

There's your ancient reptilian hypothalamus, in charge of feeding, fighting, fleeing, flocking, and fornicating.

Then there's your mammalian limbic system, in charge of hope, anxiety, love, anger, communication, cuddling—you know, chick stuff.

Then there's your bloated neocortex, in charge of philosophizing, writing biology books, and strategizing to satisfy the other two.

Over the last three hundred million years of evolution, our three distinct brains have been sloppily jury-rigged together, and they've never once agreed on anything.

When Freud made up his Superego, Ego, and Id; when Plato invented his charioteer, rational horse, and passionate horse; when the Catholic Church came up with the Father, Son, and Holy Spirit; when Clive Matson the writing teacher distinguished our internal Writer, Editor, and Crazy Child; and when Looney Tunes cartoons showed a devil on one shoulder, an angel on the other shoulder, and a head listening to both; they were elucidating our internal conflicts that come from sloppy evolutionary engineering. Now we're stuck with a Kirk, Spock, and McCoy squabbling in our skulls. To be human is to be ambivalent. You don't see lizards getting all neurotic over whether they should bite or mate. Yet I've dated people who do both at the same time.

All my neuroscientist friends tell me their colleague Paul MacLean's "triune brain" idea is simplistic. Sure, they say, evolution works with what it's already got, but it can modify those components. Reptilian parts of our brain are employed when we see color, for instance, yet reptiles don't see color the same exact way a primate can. Old brain parts get modified by new needs, just as hands for grasping trees in the jungle got modified for manipulating tools on the savanna.

Yet my dog's fear, anger, joy, and sadness are recognizable to the mammal parts in my brain that instinctively recognize these emotions. I don't bond with my dog because we have fascinating scientific debates. I bond with my dog based on the brain parts we share. All of us bond through what we have in common. Evolution has modified my body so that I cannot lick my own balls. Yet I have brain parts that can see the appeal.

So why do we watch entertainment we know is stupid? Let's look at channel surfing in neurobiological terms. Advertisers know that your ancient reptilian hypothalamus is more compelling than your mammalian limbic system, which is much more compelling than your newly-evolved neocortex.

Imagine you're an advertiser. You've paid for one minute to convince people to make an impulse purchase. Do you want to appeal to A) their urge for power and sex, B) their desire for committed emotional bonds, or do you want to C) reason with them?

Network executives. Hollywood moguls. Rock star managers.

They're all trying to capture your attention. In the competition to nab mass attention, only those who appeal to the hypothalamus survive.

I suppose Kant is compelling, in his way. But not as compelling as that Jerry Springer when they featured people who sleep with their step dads for money. I'll figure out Kant's categorical imperative later. First I want to know why that hussy think she all that . . .

Evolutionary psychology teaches that what we call shallow are actually our deepest human verities: lust, drive for prestige, vanity, envy, greed, murderous rage; as well as what we call the most profound and meaningful: love of our children, loyalty to our friends, satisfaction at a square deal, a hunger for justice, a sense of community, respect for our elders, cooperation in the pursuit of shared ideals.

If it's dramatic, it's in our genes. If you have a visceral reaction, it's because you're programmed to have a visceral reaction. If victory in the face of insurmountable odds is inspiring to you, it's because your ancestors worked together to triumph in the face of insurmountable odds again and again. All those that didn't win on long odds didn't pass on their genes.

Near-misses excite you? Chases and escapes? How about a return home after a long journey? How about a child kidnapped and then saved through heroic effort? Does the dashing stranger coming in to seduce the wife evoke any reaction in you? How about an evil tyrant who is vanquished by the oppressed villagers working together? Love torn apart by the winds of war? Consult your movie listings. They got 'em.

Is it possible to make babies corny? I don't care if it's Dickens or *All My Children*. If they throw an orphan in there, I'm weeping like an old woman. Then have some character be cruel to the orphan, and I'm ready to kill. I know it's manipulative and low-brow. I don't care. I want to see that scoundrel get his just desserts, and the orphan find a home.

Darn. Typing "find a home" just made me misty. Hang on while I dab my eyes . . .

You've got millions of years of this stuff behind you. Your body and brain were built by these dynamics. Our limbic systems were demonizing the competing tribe long before our neocortexes came to appreciate a felicitous phrase by Martin Luther King Jr. Anger is ancient and easy. Empathy for non-kin is newly evolved and hard, but it's the secret to our spectacular success.

I suppose e. e. cummings has his place. There is no doubt that poetry is hardwired in our brains. The musical use of vivid speech was the primary way culture was passed on in preliterate tribes.

But if T. S. Eliot called to your genes that same way that *Survivor* does, we wouldn't need to be forced to read him in eleventh grade. If drama calls to your genes, you volunteer to experience it. You pay nine bucks to experience it. When Spielberg makes a chase scene, you're reliving millions of years of predator/prey relationships that have built your endocrinological system. You're here because your ancestors were good at winning in the chase scenes. Spielberg is the most successful entertainer of the century, because he knows how to evoke what is universally human. I've never yet met a person who complains about pop culture who doesn't spend more time at movies than museums.

Of course, we cultural elite develop refined tastes in drama. That's why we appreciate *The Discreet Charm of the Bourgeoisie*. But there's a reason *Titanic* works in Singapore.

We like to say artistic taste is subjective. Different people like different stories. Yet the artist's pretense is that art reaches for something universal in human experience. Well, what, biologically, is universal in human experience? What behaviors does every human on the planet share, without exception?

Involuntary reflexes.

What are the eight involuntary reflexes in human communication? What are the eight genres of mass entertainment? It's written in something you can't control. It's written in your face.

20.
Let's Face It

Laugh. Weep. Gasp. Gag. Scream. Growl. Sigh. The slow gasp. You can control these about as well as you can control a sneeze. Each of these eight involuntary sounds corresponds to eight facial expressions.

The smile, the sad face, the shocked face, the disgusted face, the terrified face, the frown, the swoon, and the gape are universally understood by all humans, even children. These eight reflex facial expressions communicate eight primal emotions, and they are: happiness, sadness, surprise, revulsion, fear, anger, love, and awe. Even children born blind and deaf express all eight. Your face is like the dog's wagging tail: a reflex that subverts your choice to hide and sends emotional messages to your pack mates.

Travel with me to Papua, New Guinea and check out the Fore foragers. They will display some of the weirdest cultural practices you have ever seen (unless you live in my hometown, Berkeley). Yet you will know what a smile means, what a frown means, what surprise, horror, anger, and fear look like. No matter where you go in the world, you understand what laughter and crying mean, and every mother plays peek-a-boo with her baby.

Now go visit your local bookstore. Separated into genres are the eight universal facial expressions.

PRIMAL EMOTION	FACIAL EXPRESSION	INVOLUNTARY SOUND	GENRE OF ENTERTAINMENT
happy	smile	laugh	comedy
sad	puss face	weep	tragedy
surprise	shock	quick gasp	thriller
revulsion	disgust	gag	horror
fear	afraid	scream	ghost stories
anger	frown	growl	revenge fantasy
love	swoon	sigh	romance
awe	gape	slow gasp	magic/religion

The genres represent a taxonomy of genes for behavior. My plan is to carve out a new literary niche capturing my father's favorite: the *tsk*-and-look-askance.

The "mystery" section in the bookstore satisfies our primate curiosity to solve a puzzle. The technology in science fiction appeals to our innate fascination with novel tools. Our predictive power of anticipation, when all our senses are awakened to an approaching event, is exploited by suspense.

What, then, is "literature?" Somehow we get the sense from the keepers of the canon that genre standbys are somehow cheap, and there is some "higher" experience of art that transcends the merely visceral.

William Faulkner, in his acceptance speech for the Nobel Prize for Literature, called upon authors of the future to not write merely "for the glands." Of course, at that moment, Faulkner was being rewarded for being the best writer for the glands this country has ever known. Incest, serial killing, insanity, race war, castration, burial of the dead, biblical flood, hunting bear, rape with a corn cob— Faulkner did it all. The guy played our genome like a xylophone. Faulkner, in a suddenly noble moment, called upon writers like me to transcend the endocrinological. He didn't set the best example. What does he mean? If not for the glands, for what?

Let's check the science.

21.

Love Stinks

My mind is controlled by invisible forces. The great force controlling the urges of many animals is floating in the air. Mammals, ants, and moths all jump to the puppet strings of pheromones. You do, too.

Pheromones have no smell. The sexy scent in sweat is mostly the flatulence of bacteria, not pheromones. We *Homo sapiens* detect pheromones unconsciously. Pheromones affect (and afflict) women more than men, and women's sense of smell becomes keener during ovulation. That's why you are unaccountably attracted to that jerk. You know he's a jerk. Your friends know he's a jerk. He smells like microscopic farts. But something about him. . . .

That mysterious something is resistance to germs. Pheromones advertise our immune systems.

Claus Wedekind, a zoologist at the University of Bern in

Switzerland, wanted to figure out how fish chose mates. He wasn't satisfied with observing their behavior. He wanted to know how fish feel. He was frustrated that fish couldn't talk. He only knew of one animal that could talk. We use animals to understand human behavior, reasoned Wedekind, so why not use human behavior to understand fish?

So, to illuminate fish sex, Wedekind asked forty-four *Homo sapiens* men to wear the same T-shirt for a few nights. Men found this activity quite natural. Wedekind put each fetid T-shirt in a bag. He asked women to smell the bags, then asked them how they felt. All women were repulsed by some bags, intrigued by others. Their list of adjectives to describe the bags is unsettling. Next time you think your attraction to that guy is profound, remember these women were attracted to bags.

Suddenly nobody gave a damn about Wedekind's fish. A thousand celibate male scientists wanted to know: What's going on with the women?

A psychologist would ask them about their childhoods, but Wedekind drew blood and pulled out his microscope. It turns out that when women sniffed an immune system too similar to their own, they were grossed out. But when women sniffed an immune system that was different from their own (but not too different), it got them grinning and giggling.

"Major histocompatibility" genes play a major role in the immune systems of mammals. It turns out that female mice are more likely to get it on with males who have MHC genes most different from their own. They figure this out by smelling the male's urine.

We think of Darwinistic competition as going on among animals we can see: cheetahs, antelope, other humans. But the real war is going on inside our bodies. Possibly half the cells inside us are foreigners. We are all walking ecosystems. Germs and parasites breed much faster than big animals, and they evolve deadly warfare much quicker. So why don't they out-evolve us and kill us off like so many germs and parasites do?

The defense we have against their fast generation time is sex. Land animals that reproduce asexually can't evolve to be bigger than a slug. (Well, there is this weird whiptail lizard, but that's another story.) In the arms race between us big animals and our parasites, a versatile immune system is crucial. That's why the most attractive thing about a man is his white blood cells. Men like to look at fertile bodies. Women like to smell men's blood. (That explains half my relationships right there.) It's *literally* chemistry. Men can put a finger on what we like about the opposite sex, and women can't. That's why women think their attractions are more profound than ours. Well, ha!

A dozen studies have proved that the best thing a woman can do to cure an erratic menstrual cycle is sleep in a man's armpit. It works better than prescription drugs. The whiff of an immune system complementary to her own sends signals to her menstrual cycle that she better prepare for pregnancy, because her genes smell a healthy baby. Love really is the pits.

The creepy thing about the T-shirt study is that women who were on birth control pills found their repulsions and attractions *reversed*. Women on the pill respond to immune systems that are similar to their own and are repulsed by immune systems they would be attracted to if they were not on the pill.

Why? Because the pill prevents pregnancy by simulating the physiological symptoms of pregnancy.

The only other women who show this reversed response are

pregnant women. Pregnant women prefer the scents of immune systems similar to their own, because they need pregnancy support, and they are likely to get that from relatives. When you are pregnant, you feel the urge to be with family. Then when you are fertile again, you prefer to be around friends. When you are pregnant, scent preference is to get you support (resources). When you are fertile, scent preference is to get you sex (genes). Again we see the two separable evolutionary goals emerging in female feelings.

Guys, this is how you monitor the rhythm method: when your woman is wearing your shirt and rolling around on your pillowcase like it's chick nip, it means she's ovulating. Stay away or she'll get pregnant. When she's throwing away the sweaty socks you've left out for her enjoyment, telling you you're disgusting, and inviting her relatives over, it's safe to have sex with her. When she's in the mood, don't do it. When she's not in the mood, it's safe to do it.

This is the trouble with contraception. We are built to make more of ourselves, and anything that screws with that process screws with fundamental systems in us. No matter how hard I work at it, I can't convince my penis to enjoy wearing a condom. The dick is designed to despise all impediments to its reproductive goal. That goes for all dicks. All the activity happening down there is conspiring against us. Women trying to stick with the rhythm method still force the penis deep into their cervix at the point of male orgasm, and suck sperm into themselves at the point of their own orgasm. Nothing ruins your career plans like a pheromone.

But remember, soldiers, we're having sex to save the species. If we stop having sex, and start asexually reproducing amoeba-style, germs will make us extinct in a few generations. It doesn't take germs very long to figure out how to pick our immune system locks and eat us from within. The point of sex is to shuffle the gene deck, and we fornicate to keep those little germy bastards guessing. If you weren't already obsessed with the activity, my medical and military counsel for the human race would be: "Keep boinking! The germs are trying to pick our locks!"

Ladies, if he's got a good immune system, he doesn't need a job. The wife strategy wants resources. The concubine strategy wants healthy genes. So, go ahead. Do your duty, soldier. Sleep with the jerk.

Which reminds me of my armpit.

Ever wonder, "What's the point of underarm hair?" When you're an amateur biologist, you sit around pondering these questions. It doesn't make sense for a furless ape. Underarm hair offers no protection from the sun, it doesn't keep you warm, and it's not even visible most of the time.

I researched a study by two armpitologists, Cowley and Brooksbank. I've discovered the point of armpit hair. It's to stink. To hold onto odors. Now we know why the French are so sexy.

A lot of scientific words are just a bunch of prefixes stitched together. I actually researched a periodical called *Psychoneuroendocrinology*. Scientists just don't know how to sell themselves. They should have called it: "How the Stench of Sex Changes Your Brain." That's what that word means.

Androstenol is an aphrodisiac. It drives chicks wild. Seventy-six college students were asked to wear necklaces overnight, then filled out questionnaires about whom they had interacted with that day. Unbeknownst to the students (we writers love saying "unbeknownst"), these necklaces were laced with androstenol.

Androstenol necklaces had no effect on males. They had no effect on females' interactions with females. But the frequency and duration of females' interactions with males almost doubled over the non-necklaced, while ratings of "depth" and "personal involvement" tripled. The poor girls were trying to pair-bond with every guy they saw, having deep meaningful interactions left and right. The probability of this occurring by chance is one-quarter of a percent.

I've got good news for us guys. There are as many androstenol glands as there are hairs on the male body. Androstene glands are at the base of every male hair follicle, especially under the arm and in pubic regions. It gives off a musky odor. There's a lot of it in male urine.

Which comes in handy. The alpine ibex ram, after he out-rams all his opponents and establishes himself as alpha, dabs himself with a little yellow after-shave before he goes a'courtin' the ewes. A discriminating ewe won't choose him unless she smells victorious piss.

Guys, if you douse your body in urine, be careful. You might also seduce pigs. Exposure to androstenol makes sows assume the mating posture. Not that there's anything wrong with that. If a sow tries to mate with you, you may want to mask your scent. Many mammals accomplish this by rolling in another species' poop. But this will make you unattractive to females of your own species. You'll need more androstenol. But now we're getting into an endless loop that's hard to escape without ending up caked in crap or deflowering a pig, which is why I don't recommend the urine method for male *Homo sapiens*, unless you're a book critic.

Besides, guys, even if you choose the androstenol method, you won't get the effect you hope for. Women are not moths. They don't respond to pheromones over long distances. They have to get close. They have to stay close. Pheromones are designed to secure pair-bonds and prepare women for intercourse and ovulation. The evolutionary purpose of cuddling is in part to get the female's face in a man's armpit. But don't mention this during pillow talk.

Every time I'm chatting up a woman who keeps looking at her watch and making a face at her friends that says "rescue me," I think to myself: *If only I can find some way to get my armpit to her nose and keep it there, she will rate my conversation as deeper.*

Then I start fantasizing. Candlelight dinner. I'm sharing one of my philosophical profundities. Her voice, muffled by my armpit, is chanting, "Deeper! Deeper!"

I know the next random gift I'm getting for that cute lab technician who gives me all the data I request except her phone number: an androstenol necklace. Then we'll see who needs a shower and a job.

Every time she mentions her quote-unquote "fiancé," I wow her by reading aloud from this book. Half of women who read *Cosmopolitan* admit to infidelity. Wasn't she reading *Cosmopolitan* a moment ago?

Yet this gets me nowhere. Further research into infidelity taught me that adultery, on the surface, doesn't make much sense. Over an adulterous person's whole lifetime, almost all the sex is had with the spouse. On average, married people get a lot more sex than single people.

Hey, cool college hipster! Look at your parents! They get more sex than you!

Yet even single people have more sex with each other than adulterers have sex with secret lovers.

If married people are having most of the sex, why do men avoid commitment? That's easy. Because genetic diversity is easier to achieve if you make sperm and shoot them everywhere you can.

Okay, but if women want stable nests, why do women even bother with affairs?

Ladies, it all comes down to your orgasm. It's designed to trick you.

22.

Faked Orgasms Fool Men, but Real Orgasms Fool Women

There he is. The motorcycle guy who comes to clean your gutters. You know he's unreliable, cocky, a bad father. You know you're married to the most dependable, loving man you ever met. Yet you never go out to get the paper in your bathrobe until after he arrives. That gutter guy would be a disaster for a mate. So why does he keep strutting into your fantasies?

Blame your orgasm. It has a secret agenda.

Other female animals don't have orgasms. Okay, there's some controversy over whether rabbit and ferret females have orgasms, and the colobus monkey, stumptail macaque, and bonobo females experience some joyous orgasms. But the human female orgasm blows away even the bonobo. To reproduce, females don't need the big moment of gene propulsion, so why all the climactic fuss? Why do female *Homo sapiens* orgasm like males?

For this, let's look to the adulteresses, those wily designers of the testicle.

When good genes and resources come in the same male, that's great. It's the wife strategy all the way. When good genes come in one male, and good resources in another, the wife strategy for resources might combine with the concubine strategy for genes. It's called the adultery strategy.

Count up all the copulations in an average *Homo sapiens* adulteress's lifetime. Most of them are had with her husband. A very tiny proportion of her total sex is had with illicit lovers. Yet, one blood-type study of newborns at a British hospital accidentally discovered that 10% of babies were not fathered by the mothers' husbands! I'll never look at that row of bassinets in the nursery the same way again. A wider genetic sampling of Britons put the Milkman Effect closer to 1%, but I'm still not reassured. How does this happen?

Science has found the culprit. It's the female orgasm. Ladies, your orgasm was designed by evolution to subvert your rational plans!

Okay, fine, maybe this scientific discovery doesn't seem like such a big surprise to some of you. But how about this one? Your orgasm is a sperm-filing system. Your orgasm puts the sperm of some men over there, to the side, to be used in case of emergency, and it files the sperm of other men over here, for immediate use, to be sent straight to the ovaries, priority delivery. This filing system often completely contradicts a woman's conscious sperm-use choices. Remember, girls, once you choose multiple lovers, your orgasm has veto power.

How dare your orgasm overrule your decisions? Where does your orgasm get its balls?

Anywhere it can.

Monogamy is relatively rare in nature. Five percent of mammals are monogamous. Most of these are dogs and apes. But 92% of bird species are officially monogamous. Maybe we should look to them for example.

Look at them. Sweet lovebirds raising their little nestlings together, right next to the happy nests of their next-door neighbors. Talk about family values! We want them to stay healthy, don't we? Let's take a blood test.

Wolfgang Forstmeier, a German ornithologist, ran some routine DNA tests on newborn dusky warblers and revealed that 45% weren't sired by the female's mates, but by next-door neighbors.

The hussies! How could they? Ask female genes. Once long chickling childhoods meant males evolved to care for the females' nests, females realized they didn't have to get good genes and good resources in the same male. They could "marry" the male with good nesting and food-finding talents, yet secretly get knocked up by those sexy bad boys with the longer, more colorful tails. So while her husband is home baby-sitting, she is out cuckolding him. The females are so good at this secrecy, they even fooled the ornithologists, who didn't know the illicit boinking was going on until they did the DNA tests.

This trampy strategy led to the evolution of a competing strategy in the male: paranoia. When he's not baby-sitting the eggs or chicks, he darts around spying on his mate, herding her around, chirping out his territory, and dive-bombing any hapless male who flits within flirting range. Every time the harried cuckold stops for a rest, the female ducks behind a bush for a quickie with one of the big-tailed males. Sure it's scandalous, but she has her future chicks to consider. She's got the resources. Now she needs the best genes.

Biologists call this the "sexy son strategy." Once some arbitrary quality like colorful tails comes to be seen as sexy, mating with sexy males will create more sexy males, and sexiness will do the genes good over the next generations. It's a phenomenon that feeds off itself and creates bad boy birds cruising around looking for gutters to clean out while the husband is off at work gathering worms.

The "sexy son strategy" runs rampant in nature. Female side-blotched lizards, given a choice between the best bodies and the best shelters, will chose a mate with a small body if he has the largest territory and the most baby-protecting rocks.

But that is a wife strategy for resources. For the best genes, a concubine strategy comes in handy. One group of male side-blotchers court females by displaying their large homes. Another group courts them by doing push-ups. Though female side-blotchers marry the wealthy males, they secretly mate with the buff males. These females have a special talent for reserving sperm, yet they do it without all the orgasmic hoopla. Sperm gotten from bad boy males is used to make bad boy baby males. Sperm gotten from property-owning males is used to make daughters.

Why? Because females who pair-bond usually want sizable territories where resources are plentiful for the hatchlings. But the "sexy son strategy" pops up in many species. Secret sex with sexy males will produce sexy sons who will seduce future females. Making males is a high-risk game. Sons can breed a whole lot or not at all. Females can't spread genes the way males can, but they can through their sons, which makes females adopt the occasional high-risk male behavior and have an affair with a sexy male. The tension in pair-bonding females remains: responsible resource provider or sexy bad boy?

Preferential sperm-treatment goes on inside the adulterous

females of many pair-bonded species. Culture matters, of course. Among red-wing blackbird cultures that are morally deprived, 18% of females' copulations are adulterous, and 48% of the nestlings are born from adulterous matings. Among red-wing blackbird cultures that are morally upright, 6% of female copulations are adulterous, and 23% of nestlings are born from adulterous matings.

Even red-wing blackbird females whose husbands have vasectomies are managing miraculous conceptions! (I want to meet the graduate student who gives a bird a vasectomy. For this his mother sent him to college?)

Both permissive and prudish bird wives are finding ways to favor adulterous genes. We don't know how they manage this, but we know why.

Remember the T-shirt study? Bluethroat females are mostly monogamous, but the chicklings sired by adulterous lovers have more active immune systems than those sired with their husbands. (Maybe we should try the T-shirt study on bluethroat females—if only we could get the males to wear little shirts.) We see the pattern again: marry for resources, mate for genes.

But everybody knows birds are flighty, and lizards are flaky! Surely, we higher apes don't reject sperm deposited by our husbands and favor sperm deposited by our secret lovers! Do we?

Chimpanzee females are all proud concubines. They mate like a lady chimpanzee should: promiscuously and publicly. But there is a less common mating strategy: trysts. Even though a female mates with many males, with the dominant males getting extra, sometimes she will favor one particular low-status male, and actually sneak off with him to have *private* sex together. Judging by the outrage, many chimps believe private sex is an abomination in the eyes of God. It's hard not to see their trysts as romantic, and it's hard not to call them lovers. These consort-ships, though rare, can actually result in more pregnancies. By one measurement, secret chimp affairs resulted in only 2% of the boinkings, yet DNA tests showed they resulted in 50% of the offspring!

So, even though females received twenty-five times more copulations from their many "husbands," half their babies were fathered by their few "lovers."

If the male chimps got access to this data, they might acquire some much-needed perspective. No matter how male chimps compete with each other for extra sex, female chimps still find ways to get the genes they want. Maybe males should spend less time fighting each other and more time courting females.

But that's not all. Though a quarter of all sex was had by dominant males who were guarding their mates and beating up interlopers, three-quarters of the sex was had by just about anybody. Nevertheless, most of the remaining 50% of offspring were fathered by dominant males. So let's look at the stats:

Seventy-three percent of the sex was a free-for-all, and it resulted in very few offspring.

Twenty-five percent of the sex was with the dominant male, and it resulted in almost half the offspring.

Two percent of the sex was romantic and secret, and it resulted in half the offspring.

This means chimp chicks are using some power of contraception. Whether it's through the rhythm method, something akin to orgasm, or her emotional state during sex that affects her hormones, a female chimp is able to prevent pregnancy from three-quarters of her matings.

What we are seeing here is a dual favoritism. Female chimps want the sperm of powerful males. Females also want the sperm of males with whom they are more intimate. Females definitely do not want the sperm of just anybody.

This means that females are using at least 75% of their sex for social manipulation. Unbeknownst to the male orgiasts, the free-for-all sex is not for procreation. Her sluttiness has a social strategy. Can you blame her? No particular male chimp is the paragon of fatherhood, but all of them together protect and play with the off-spring enough. They also have a nasty habit of killing infants they don't know. You need a bunch of male chimps to make one decent father, so the female chimp has sex with all of them. That way each male looks at the youngsters of all the females he's had sex with and feels a vague fatherly protectiveness.

And take a look at the sperm output from your average big-balled chimp. Females must walk around with much of their body weight in sperm. When it comes to sperm-filing systems, female chimps have a whole bureaucracy in there. Sluttiness is a strategy that best serves females: keep the males competing, have sex with all of them, use only the best sperm, get all of them to baby-sit your children. When you're a mother chimp with several hus-bands, having sex is a full-time job. Never underestimate female power. No alpha male could ever hope to manipulate so many apes at once.

But don't give yourself too much credit, primate females. You don't need to be that smart to outwit a male using sex. I'm sure you don't consider lemmings all that smart. Yet lady lemmings have sex with as many males as they can. And it ain't for their sperm. Sex not only makes babies, it saves babies. One male lemming killed 42% of the babies of females who didn't have sex with him. So females have sex with every male, so every male thinks maybe all the kids are his. Duh.

But, surely, we humans don't shift sperm around inside our hips like we're dancing a mambo! We make rational choices!

Right?

Ladies, let's use evolutionary biology to find out what your unconscious tricks you into choosing.

23.

You Don't Have an Orgasm, an Orgasm Has You

A research project measured the amount of bare flesh exposed by females dancing at nightclubs. (These are *Homo sapiens* females, by the way.) The researchers noticed the amount of flesh exposed varied cyclically. At certain times of the month, little flesh was exposed. At other times of the month, lots of flesh was exposed. The researchers asked the women when they were having their periods. It was discovered the women were unconsciously choosing skimpier outfits when they were ovulating.

Oh, stop trying to act like you're so pure, female mammals. At ovulation time, female rats are willing to crawl over an electric fence to reach a mate. I know a few female *Homo sapiens* who have put themselves through even more pain to get their paws on a male.

If you think your wily female unconscious stops at choosing your wardrobe, you're in for a big surprise.

When you're a guy like me, and you see a book called *Human Sperm Competition: Copulation, Masturbation, and Infidelity*, you pick it up. Those are my three main interests and one main hobby right there. The book only confused me more. How am I supposed to figure women out when they can't even figure themselves out? Some women don't know where their clitoris is. Others don't know when they ovulate.

Yet they don't need to know. Unfaithful wives unconsciously favor their lovers during ovulation. A study of 3,679 women in Britain revealed that wives are more likely to cheat during the four days they are most fertile, and more likely to have simultaneous orgasms while they are cheating. This finding really opened the floodgates on vagina studies.

If female lizards, birds, and chimps can evolve their own special method of sperm allocation, why can't we? It's called "the female orgasm."

Here's how it works. A woman's orgasm can either block sperm or suck sperm deeper inside. It depends on how you time it. If a woman orgasms more than one minute before male ejaculation, her orgasm will block his sperm. If she orgasms just before the male ejaculates, she is sucking sperm toward her ovaries.

But men usually orgasm either too soon or even more too soon. Who can predict? Don't worry, girls, you don't need to be psychic. Mother Nature has provided you with a backup plan. If your guy orgasms first, you must orgasm within forty-five minutes to suck sperm deeper inside. If you wait forty-five minutes, then orgasm, you're blocking his sperm again.

Guys, enter her bed with a stopwatch and find out how much

she likes you. Simultaneous orgasms mean that not only does the female like you, her orgasms like you. It's hard to get them to agree, but it's easier to achieve impregnation if you seduce both. If she orgasms too soon or too late, she doesn't want your sperm, she wants your support.

Okay, husbands. Brace yourselves for this scientific discovery. Are you sitting down? Here goes:

Women's orgasms with adulterous lovers typically retain three times as much sperm as orgasms with husbands. Maybe this has something to do with why, when you haven't seen your wife in a few days, you ejaculate three times as much sperm as normal. Sex with husbands serves primarily to maintain bonds. Sex with secret lovers serves primarily to get genes, and secondarily to forge bonds with a possible replacement husband.

Why don't you husbands stop reading here and glare paranoiacally at your wife?

Are you back? Good. Don't panic. Women want monogamy because they want to feel special. A woman's orgasm rate is twice as high in a monogamous relationship as in an open relationship, and her orgasm rate is four to five times higher with a husband than when she's single. However, wives are more likely to cheat when they ovulate, and orgasms retain more adultery sperm than married sperm. So, judging by the Orgasmagraph, women are least orgasmic when they are not made to feel special, more orgasmic in a monogamous relationship, and especially orgasmic when married— though women are most productively orgasmic when committing adultery.

And remember, how orgasmic a woman is when she has sex does not necessarily have anything to do with how often she wants to have sex. Some women want more sex before marriage than after marriage, and most women want more sex as they approach fifty, but how a woman's sexual desire changes day to day and throughout her life is another story that will require several volumes. How a man's sex drive changes through his life can be summed up in a haiku:

Before thirty-five,
My dick woke up before me.
Now my dick sleeps in.

What's significant about sperm competition, the wardrobe choices of females, and the timing of female orgasms, is that it is all going on without conscious awareness. It's just happening. A husband's sperm can increase in numbers and compete with a lover's sperm without the husband knowing the other lover exists. Females choose a style of clothes because that's the way they feel that day, not because they rationally want to get pregnant by a stranger they might meet that particular ovulation night. We have all wondered why orgasm happens and why it doesn't, and we all try to control it with varying success. But it's not really up to us. When it comes to our genes' reproductive agendas, what feels to us like conscious choices might actually be the marionette strings of our biology.

Men have similar problems trying *not* to orgasm. His mammal brain's agenda: hang on a little longer to please his elusively orgasming woman to maintain their pair-bond. His reptilian orgasm's agenda: pair-bond, shmair-bond; get sperm in there quick.

Male orgasm has been around a lot longer than deep relationships. The tension between his orgasm and her orgasm should be equivalent to the tension between his fear of commitment and her cautiousness about consummation. That's why in order to orgasm, some women need to concentrate, and some men, to put off orgasm, need to think about something else. My method is to list each Yankee baseball player's batting average. The second a man thinks about what he's *actually doing*, it's over. So the only way a man can enjoy sex is to not think about what he's doing. Can you blame us if we extend this strategy to relationships?

Now we know why our instincts think they're smarter than our rational brains. They've been around longer. Even geckos experience sexual attractions that were structured by their ancestral environments, and they manage to mate and rear babies without the foggiest clue what they're doing. They do things because they want to do things, not because they've figured it out. Our mating behaviors worked just fine long before our neocortical calculations came along. I hate to break it to you, but our base instincts have much longer track records for survival than our high-flung ideas. Our reptilian brains set up veto power before they installed our neocortexes.

I have a friend who's in love. She's a biochemist genius. She got perfect scores on all the science geek tests. She's so smart, she can tell you all about her scientific discoveries without using a single understandable word. Yet when she talks about her guy, she says things like, "Did you see how he put mustard on his sandwich? I mean, mustard! That's so him!"

That's her orgasm talking. Geniuses in love act like morons because their noses have picked up pheromones from an immune system complementary to their own. Their reptile brains have decided this is The One, and their human neocortexes will do all they can to rationalize why mustard is romantic. When your genes need you to breed, the last thing they want is you thinking clearly.

The neocortex was designed to help you socially strategize among people you don't want to make babies with. If your nose tells you your immune system perfectly complements the immune system of the village idiot, your genes don't want your brain figuring out that this spells social suicide. The biological function of love is to make you passionate, impulsive, and stupid. That's why it feels so good. Notice how lizards don't fall in love. They don't need to. They're already stupid.

Remember, ladies: Hot for the power suit? That's a wife strategy for resources. Hot for the immune system? That's a concubine strategy for genes.

This is how we should look at the double-mating strategies of men and women. We don't do things because we want to spread our genes. We want to do things because those actions spread our ancestor's genes. Females don't consciously decide to strategize for one man's resources and another man's genetic material. Female feelings are structured by biology to strategize for optimum sperm and optimum nests. Two reproductive goals—one to create offspring, one to raise offspring—will select for two behavior strategies. If both resources and genes come in the same male, that's fine. If not, fantasies arise.

Too bad that understanding where our desires come from does not justify acting on them. No biological explanation for how the urge to murder was constructed by natural selection will ever justify murder. Just because an action paid off reproductively for our ancestors does not make it morally right.

Natural does not mean good. Disease is natural. Murder, rape, lying, and adultery are all quite natural, as are love, compassion, trust, and loyalty. The gene is so amoral, it constructed both morality and immorality to serve itself. Darwinian selection gave us a suite of emotions, among them love and murderous rage. It did not tell us what actions to choose.

Who is that knocking? It's the gutter guy come to collect his payment. Your bird-brain just told you to open your robe before you open the door. Your human neocortex says inhibit that instinct and don't risk losing your precious pair-bond.

Free genes are waiting at your door. The size of your husband's testicles tells you some of your female ancestors succeeded with the adultery strategy. The average size ratio of men and women tells you some of your male ancestors succeeded by killing or humiliating other men.

The wail of your imminent orgasm tells you sluttiness sometimes paid off. The surge in your heart tells you faithfulness sometimes paid off.

Which do you choose?

24.

Why Your Clitoris Is Hard to Find

No man ever visited a sex therapist with the lament, "I've never had an orgasm, and I don't know where my penis is!"

Why do *Homo sapiens* females have hidden clitorides? (Yes, that's the plural for "clitoris.") They are so hidden, in fact, some *Homo sapiens* females can't even find their own. Why does Mother Nature make it difficult to please women?

Consider the biological riddle:

The penis and the male orgasm. Both very important to reproduction. The penis is easy to find, the male orgasm easy to achieve.

The clitoris and the female orgasm. They wouldn't have evolved if they weren't important to reproduction. Yet the clitoris is like the Loch Ness Monster: there are legends and some fuzzy photographs, a few dedicated spelunkers *claim* to have glimpsed it, but basically you gotta have faith. And attaining the female orgasm is like trying to attain nirvana.

Not that hiding your genitals is a bad idea. Most African predators have penises and testes that are tiny and tucked away like valuable jewelry. The genitals are always protected beneath the animal, in the back, where they can't be bitten off.

But the penis on the upright *Homo sapiens* is extravagantly visible, with a tuft of hair calling attention to the spot, exposed right about the height of a hyena's teeth. Like a peacock's tail, it seems to scream: "Nyah, nyah, predators! Bite this!" Why is the most sensitive and reproductively valuable part of a *Homo sapiens* male waving out there in the wind?

Biology tells us why: because women like them. Women's choice sculpted the male penis the same way peahen choice designed the peacock's tail. Whatever females enjoy in mates keeps getting built to please females.

Well, I like giving women orgasms. Why hasn't male choice had any effect on making women's clitorides more prominent? When I'm trying to get a woman to like me, I don't want an Easter egg hunt. Why can't anything ever be simple with women?

Don't look to the field of psychology for answers. Men have been so clueless about the clitoris that Sigmund Freud, generally considered a man of deep insight, developed a whole theory about why vaginal orgasm is superior to clitoral orgasm. I feel sorry for Mrs. Freud.

Don't look to women, either. Years of interrogating women never got me anywhere. Girlfriends got irritated, and women I met on the bus got alienated. It ain't easy conducting a scientific survey. I literally had to do academic research before I understood what the clitoris was, where it was, and how it worked. Thank goodness for *The Hite Report.*

It's not fair. Women don't need to consult anatomy maps to locate my penis. After the movies and dinners and pretending I give a damn about Oprah and all that time on the couch, why do I have to go on a safari through a labial labyrinth?

Only women would have a locus of pleasure so obscure it's called the "G-spot." You know why it's called the "G-spot?" Because you have to try spots A through F and H through Z before you find it. Just remember it's about three inches in, and straight up. Maybe this is why men are good with directions. Tests in cognitive spatial abilities show that men think in abstract maps, while women go straight for the landmarks.

Imagine a scavenger hunt through New York: Men have to find (by feel) an object just under the lid of a manhole above the Lincoln Tunnel, then crawl in and find another invisible spot hidden on the roof of the dark underground cavern. Women have to find the Empire State Building. Ready? Go!

I think it's fair to say this race is rigged, and Mother Nature most definitely is not a guy. The Grafenberg Spot is named after a man, and we men should recognize Grafenberg as the Columbus of subterranean exploration.

Next time you have sex with a woman, bring this book as a guide. Start by inserting your finger, palm facing up, then make a come-hither motion. The aroused G-spot feels like a spongy walnut. The G-spot is analogous to the male's prostate, so every woman has one. For G-spot orgasm during intercourse, it helps if the woman gets on top, puts her hands behind her heels, and leans way back. (If you're under 18, please skip the preceding paragraph.)

Female orgasm would not have evolved if female pleasure wasn't vital to attaining pregnancy and securing pair-bonds. So why not make it easy for men? Put the female pleasure-button on the end of a long flesh stick that pokes out proudly for all to see!

Okay, I guess that would be a penis, so scratch that idea, but this is the type of design Nature provides for male genitals all the time. The mandrill has a bright red penis, bright yellow tip, and lilac-colored scrotum. Why not make the female clitoris fluorescent green?

Vervet monkeys have red penises, white pubic hair, and blue scrotums. Forget the bald eagle. This monkey's red, white, and blue display is more the message we want an American mascot to send.

When I get aroused, I can't hide it. How about when the female gets aroused, a flag shoots up from her vagina saying: "Ready!" Or rockets shoot from her crotch?

European men 450 years ago strutted their stuff in decorated codpieces (British for jock strap). Hulu warriors paint their faces in all the colors of a primate scrotum: cheeks bright yellow, eyes red, and beards blue. In many hunter-gatherer tribes, men wear giant extensions on their penises. New Guinean chiefs wear perpetually upright "penis sheaths" that are tall enough to reach their useless nipples. Just in case women aren't getting the hint, they organize penis parades. Men provide this service for free. How come chicks never do that?

Admittedly, females do have a tuft of hair calling attention to the reproductive area. This gets men's attention. Oh, they are so good at getting men's attention: oversized breasts, round hips, soft skin, an instinct for adornment, batty eyelashes, a certain walk. But from there it stops being clear. Why do *Homo sapiens* females have so many body parts designed to get men's attention, yet so few to instruct men how to get them off?

In fact, if you look at the history of our pelvis evolution, you can see a steady trend toward deeper vaginas, which required longer penises, which favored yet deeper vaginas, which continues to make penises even longer. Pretty soon, getting an erection will mean a slap in the face—*by your penis*. Why are ovaries running away from us? Are they trying to burrow up into woman's brain? (That would explain a few things.) Do women want babies or don't they? What's with all the hide-and-seek with female anatomy?

To develop a scientific theory for pleasing a woman, the last thing you want to do is just ask a woman. This is not a route we male theorists traditionally take. If you don't see why, tap the nearest woman on the shoulder, and say, "Excuse me, how do you like your clitoris to be stimulated? This is a scientific study, so please use visual aids." My prediction is she won't contribute to the advancement of science—not so long as the female's biological need for coyness is in place. To uncover the Deep Mystery of Women, there's only one guru you can turn to: an amateur male biologist.

Ready? Here goes.

The female clitoris is all about us, the men. No, I'm not saying that just because it fits in well with every other sex theory men have ever produced. I'm speaking as a biologist here.

The function of the hidden clitoris is to judge how good a lover the male is.

Think about it from the female genes' perspective. If the clitoris just hung out there penis-style, it would be easily located and stimulated, and, like a penis, it would be more prone to make its owner pursue intercourse. But females are designed, body and soul, to be more choosy. Female pleasure is something that has to be earned. By making the clitoris hard to find, Mother Nature is making sure females choose the most seductive men.

First, it helps the "sexy son strategy." By mating with the best lovers, she produces sons who are the best at pleasing women, who will then grow up to seduce more women and pass on more good lover genes. When women choose a mate, they have their future women to consider.

Then it helps the "pair-bond strategy." Sex serves to make babies, but sexuality serves to rear babies. The hidden mysteries of ovulation, the clitoris, and female emotions are designed to entice *Homo sapiens* males for lifelong baby-sitting and provisioning. It really helps males evolve attachment and intuition if women are difficult to seduce.

This is why women are more prone to foreplay and reluctant to have intercourse, and why men complain that women are teasing them. Female emotions are structured to test the male's ability to please women, as well as his willingness to invest labor, tenderness, and fierce protection in her babies. They want to see the man work, they want to see a little tenderness, and expressing a killer instinct at the right moment doesn't hurt. It's a tall order, and indiscriminate orgasming is not going to get the woman anywhere. Her body wants to test if he has good women-pleasing genes, and good fathering genes. After all, isn't that the function of men?

The Penis Principle is easy to grasp: penises deposit plentiful sperm and women like them. Thus they have been under selection pressure to get bigger and easy to notice.

The Clitoris Principle requires us to probe a little deeper: clitorides produce orgasms that pull plentiful sperm toward the rare eggs. It's always in a rare egg's interests to make plentiful sperm compete for them. Thus clitorides have been under selection pressure to remain small, hidden, and a challenge to males.

Look at the nearest erect penis. If you're a fertile female, there's probably one nearby. It's not exactly subtle, is it? The male goal is complicated only to the extent that the female complicates it. When childhoods are long, it is in Mother Nature's interest that egg-makers always remain a little more elusive. By remaining mysterious, females make males work harder, creating continued selection pressure for more sensitive and parental males.

A predictable woman is not a sexy woman. A mysterious woman is a sexy woman. This is why women drive men crazy, both in the good way and the bad way. It is not in an egg-maker's interest to be "figured out." The clitoris and female psychology are designed to stay just out of reach, just a little teasing, so a man will bond through sexuality, fall in love, and stick around to raise the offspring. In our species, female choice caused the evolution of men's deep intuition of women's feelings.

You scoff, ladies? Would you rather have sex with a baboon male? Baboon males don't spend all their time trying to "figure females out." They'd rather fight than father. Just because *Homo sapiens* male's empathizing skills are not up to female standards doesn't mean they don't out-feminine male baboons. Many male *Homo sapiens* gain weight when their mate gets pregnant, their estrogen goes up, and some experience ghost labor contractions and even morning sickness. This sissy behavior evolved through your mate choices, ladies.

When it's up to the *Homo sapiens* female, nobody gets inside her palace without ringing her doorbell. The heights of pleasure *Homo sapiens* females are capable of reaching show us how important women's choice was on the Pleistocene savanna. There's lots of other evidence, too: the inconvenient size of the penis, the merely moderate size difference in males and females, the tiny fangs on men, the similarity of brains, the deep connection men forge with their mates and offspring—all speak of the evolutionary power of female choice. Among hominids, there was a lot more courting than there was kidnapping. Romance was more common than rape. Dads were more common than deadbeats. Crucial to human evolution was men bringing women to heights of pleasure, and crucial to the evolution of humane males was women choosing less violent, more maternal males.

Hot sex. Peace. Romantic love. We owe it all to the clitoris, hidden ovulation, and feminine emotional complexity.

This is the situation, and we males are stuck with it.

But there is a deeper mystery: why is there a plural for clitoris? In what circumstance would somebody need to say, "Okay, ladies, let's move those clitorides this way." If women invented this plural, why don't they ever say it around me? If a man invented this plural, what's his technique and does he give lessons? I would love to be in a situation where I get to refer to multiple clitorides.

There are many linguistic mysteries concerning the sexes. One was introduced to me by my fellow amateur biologist: George Carlin. I attended his presentation at my college. After decades of anthropological and lexicographic research, Carlin was ready to present his list of men's slang words for masturbation. He went on and on. The audience remained scientifically attentive. After twenty minutes, he stopped.

Then he listed women's slang phrases for masturbation. There were only two. One of them was "making soup." Carlin assured us that this was fully researched, and he announced that if anybody knew of a third slang term for female masturbation, to please inform him.

Why do men have thousands of phrases for choking the chicken, while women have two phrases for making chicken soup for your soul? Does it have something to do with women's coyness and men's display?

This will require a more penetrating analysis. Nietzsche was trying to be cynical when he said: "For woman, man is the means. The child is the end." Of course, Nietzsche was no better. He eventually went insane from the syphilis he probably caught in a whorehouse while he was manfully pursuing anonymous sex as a means to the end of children.

And what was a high-minded philosopher like Nietzsche doing in a whorehouse? How come women weren't paying *him* for sex?

25.

March of the Penguin Prostitutes

Male hominids turned the fact that they make lots of sperm and don't get pregnant to their advantage. Female hominids turned the fact that males desperately compete for rare eggs to female advantage.

When you're the one with a womb and breasts, that's a competitive disadvantage. But when sperm are worthless, and eggs are precious, and you're the one holding the eggs, that's a competitive advantage. Females have their vulnerability, and they have their bargaining chip.

Consider penguin prostitutes. Male Adelie penguins pay for sex with rocks. Don't laugh. Imagine what a penguin would think if he saw a female *Homo sapiens* trade sex for some colored pieces of paper.

Rocks are a valuable currency among Adelie penguins. These birds breed in mud. This may sound sexy to you, but it's a terrible way to raise chicks. Rocks are rare, yet females need them to construct a high and dry platform for their nests. And we all know what happens to males when there is a resource females need. Males fight for rocks, steal them, hoard them, and display them. Females pair-bond with good rock-providers. When a husband penguin leaves the nest for work, he's out to earn rocks to bring home for their nest. That must be why penguins evolved to look like they're wearing business suits.

But sometimes when the hubby isn't looking, the wife slips out of the nest to earn some extra rocks the ancient way. Sashaying the way only a penguin can sashay, she approaches the rock nest of a bachelor penguin. Like a typical male, his rock home is less of a nest than a pile. She does the standard dip of the head and coy askance glance. If he responds with the universal gawk of the horny male, she waltzes in, lays on her back, and spreads her flippers. Biologists have gathered enough data and crunched enough numbers to establish that this is an invitation to mate. He gets his rocks off, she gets a rock. She takes a stone from the john penguin's pad and waddles back to her nest with it. Hubby comes home from work and never seems to notice anything different about his wife. Luckily, penguins don't have much range in their facial expressions.

In the 1980's, the National Survey of Sexual Attitudes and Lifestyles quizzed British and French people about the lifetime number of opposite-sex partners they've had. In England, men averaged ten and women averaged three-and-a-half. In France, men averaged eleven and women averaged three-and-a-half. This can't be right, because men and women need each other for each heterosexual boink, so they should average the same. Yet 1% of straight men claim more than 100 partners! Is everybody lying?

The European survey did not take prostitution into account. In the U.S.A., one in 5000 women is a prostitute. Prostitutes average roughly 600 clients per year, and some of the harder working girls have more than 10,000 partners a year (which is, like, thirty clients a day)! That means two out of every 10,000 women in the U.S.A. are having sex with most of the guys who solicit prostitution. When you factor in American prostitution with the European numbers, the average number of partners for men and women miraculously becomes much closer to equal. Most women average a little more than three partners in a lifetime, yet a minuscule proportion of women approach 1000 per year. Our conclusion? Most of the Don Juans who claim more than 100 conquests are paying for it.

Across all cultures, *Homo sapiens* males pay for prostitution far more than females. The statistically small minority of females who pay for sexual relations typically require deeper connections with their prostitutes. Surveys suggest more talking, more time spent together, more sharing of personal life, more cuddling. A male prostitute I interviewed expressed his mystification that many women pay hundreds of dollars just to be listened to. Yet men are paying their prostitutes to not talk. Whether you are the one who makes rare eggs, or you are the one who makes plentiful sperm, natural selection will structure your desires accordingly.

In general, though not universally, females are less capable of separating sex and emotional bonds, while males—in general, but not universally—are able to enjoy sex with emotional bonds and sex without a word exchanged.

Though we should keep in mind that some men report feeling lonely after anonymous sex, many men describe emotionally attached sex and emotionally unattached sex as two separate and unrelated experiences.

Though some women report they enjoy sex with strangers, far more report feeling "dirty" and "used" after anonymous sex.

Remember, ladies, he can have anonymous no-feelings sex because his sperm are worthless. Mother Nature gave women deep emotions with regards to sex because their eggs are precious. Female emotions are structured to protect eggs. Male emotions are structured to give away free sperm.

Oh, but don't worry. Mother Nature cursed men with intense feelings to protect their reproductive interests as well. If you want to discover what they are, sleep with your guy's best friend.

26.

Free Love Causes War

I used to be one of those non-monogamous free-and-easy California guys. George Bush Sr. referred to us as that "hot tub crowd." I knew my ideals. Love should be free. Sex should be non-exclusive. Possessive passion was an oxymoron. Before our pornotopia came to an end with all the screaming and hair-pulling of a chimp riot, I was living the carefree life of an alpha gorilla. I was even a vegetarian.

I had one primary relationship. My girlfriend was okay with me sleeping with my harem. In fact, as my closest confidant, she wanted to hear all the intimate details. It wasn't until I started to confide our intimate details to another women that she put on a big display in my kitchen, hurling much of my glassware and hitting all the high notes I thought only an enraged chimpette could hit.

I was disdainful. What was her problem? Didn't she know that possessiveness was primitive, man? Surely she didn't think intimacy should be restricted, that my trust was something she *owned*.

After all, wasn't I okay with her having intimate friendships with many of our male friends? I loved her, so of course I was open-minded about her getting yet more love. I didn't mind if she confided our intimate details. She could brag about my prowess as much as she wanted! We idealists had a responsibility to expand the circle of peace and harmony, and my fellow males should not be excluded.

It wasn't until she actually slept with one of them that I felt the overwhelming urge to bash my hippie-friend's skull with a big club. I wasted no time facing off with my rival on his front lawn territory, baring my canines and puffing out my chest. We hooted and shoved and stamped, then grabbed each other by our ponytails. It was the clash of the sensitive New Age guys.

Our entire hot tub tribe spontaneously switched our ideals from peace and love to war and hate. Nasty secrets got exposed at full volume. Hippie-chicks grabbed each other's beads and tried to garrote each other. One guy who'd fathered a love-child with another woman got hit upside the head with the business end of maternal instincts. Our commune went the way of communism. It Chernobyled itself.

Sex and intimacy is not some gift from the universe designed to make us happy. Sex and intimacy is an expensive responsibility constructed by life-and-death competition on the Pleistocene savanna, and our glands are booby-traps triggered to go off when somebody enhances or threatens our reproductive interests. Apes with long childhoods are innately designed to take a proprietary interest in their mates. If you are indifferent to someone, you set him free. If you love someone, you try to possess him.

Our choice of words belies our true feelings: "my" husband, "my" wife, "my" kid. My genetic interests are the same as me. Love isn't free. Love is expensive.

Jealous males sired more children than tolerant males. In our species, males who hated being cuckolded, who murdered other males who mated with their mates, passed on more genes than those who were fine with their mates accepting sperm donations from other men. When it comes to wombless apes, jealousy causes either vigilance or violence.

If this weren't always true for our species, men and women would not be moderately different sizes, men would not have an instinct for ambition, and females would not develop an attraction to ambition. Nor would the most common cause of homicide worldwide be trivial insults to male pride. Public insults to male honor mean a dip in status, and status is what gets a Pleistocene man sex. To men, sometimes lethal violence is preferable to accepting insult. Marvin Wolfgang interviewed convicted murderers in Philadelphia, categorized twelve motives, and reported that almost 40% were caused by an "altercation of relatively trivial origin: insult, curse, jostling, etc."

Cut your caveman some slack. When his head swivels for any anonymous pair of buttocks, when his temper flares over imagined slights to his machismo, that's his primate brain talking, remembering the harem-hoarding days when anonymous buttocks and male hierarchies meant life or death. Pride and promiscuity (also the title of a Jane Austen spoof I recommend) seems stupid only in modern society. Pride and promiscuity were smart male reproductive strategies long before our ancestors climbed out of the seas, lost their fins, and learned to discuss where to meet for coffee. Our brand-new neocortexes, built recently by sociality and language, are only a thin overlay on top of our ancient animal brains. The purpose of our neocortexes is to control our instincts for long-term planning in a social context. Yet the point of rationality is to serve instincts. Without instinct, rationality has no point.

There is a film of Steve Ballmer, chief executive of Microsoft, circulating on the internet. He's giving a speech to his underlings. It was entitled "Monkey Boy." Because of our jealousy instincts concerning people who have earned higher status than we have, we all enjoy humiliating rich and famous people, so let's give old Ballie a ribbing. When you read the transcript of his address, you hear an entrepreneur exhorting his employees to uphold the Microsoft ideals of diligence and innovation. But when you watch the film without sound, you see an alpha ape displaying. Ballmer marches around the stage waving his arms and making faces that look distinctly simian. His neocortex, in charge of language and analysis, is making an inspiring speech. His body language, controlled by his primate limbic system, is saying, "I am the alpha male! I will mount any female I want! Hoo! Hoo! Hoo! Ah! Ah! Ah!" There are moments when he looks like he's throwing invisible feces.

I'm sure I never did that. I made a perfectly scholarly argument proving why I was entitled to multiple mates, while my girlfriend must preserve her purity except in the case of me. It's not that I was jealous of our comrade, Moonglow, per se, it's that he didn't tell me about the sex before it happened, which is the same as lying, in the Heideggerian sense. It's an intricate philosophical position that takes a large male brain to understand. I recommended she read Foucault. Her pointing out that I was marching in circles and waving my fork like a rainforest frond was no measure of some deep primitive instinct that was dictating my philosophy to me. Moonglow betrayed the ideology, that is the problem. The rational thing to do was to crush Moonglow's skull with my lava lamp and dress my woman in a tie-dye burka. It was for her own protection! Why couldn't she understand that?

Among marmoset monkeys, slutty males produce more surviving offspring than monogamous males, because they spread more sperm around. But the females who mate with these cads have fewer surviving offspring than females who mate with monogamous males, because promiscuous males provide less childcare. That's the tension in male and female interests. Even if long childhoods make male and female behaviors more alike, polygyny is always better for the genes of a sperm-maker, and monogamy is always better for the genes of a womb-carrier. (Except when she wants to sneak in some bad boy genes.)

In many societies that allow men to have multiple wives, children of these marriages are less likely to survive than children of monogamous marriages, and second and third wives have fewer surviving children than first wives. Yet men with extra wives have more children overall. Having lots of wives is reproductively good for a man. Being one among many wives is not good for a woman. Needless to say, co-wives don't always get along, and most divorces in polygynous societies are attributed to wives fighting. (Because polygynous men, to judge from their own reports, are faultless saints.)

In specific cases, women will happily share a rich husband and become best friends. Why aren't these women jealously fighting? Sharing a husband is only reproductively beneficial for a woman when the ratio of male wealth to number of dependents is low— meaning the man has enough wealth for twenty wives and families but only has ten. That way the husband's wealth is not spread too thin. These well-provided-for women—whether they be Mormon or Pakistani or Aleut—often bond amongst themselves and boss the alpha male around. They form a united front and exhibit no signs of jealousy. The anthropologist Laura Betzig put it best when she asked women plainly: Which would you rather be, the third wife of John F. Kennedy or the first wife of Bozo the Clown?

But we broke guys can get extra wives, too. Fellahs, are you sick and tired of your possessive Western woman who is so narrow-minded about you sleeping with her sister? There are more open-minded societies where we paupers can fulfill all our fantasies. In these places, several nubile, naked women volunteer to share one man's genitalia and cook for him. If you want to live in a place where women recommend your penis to their friends, go to a place where you can catch lots of lethal diseases. All you have to do to live a porn star life is walk naked among Tsetse flies and drink from streams where sick children defecate and die. If you reach adulthood without crippling deformities, grotesque boils, or dropping dead, you'll get extra sex!

In societies where disease runs rampant, women sometimes prefer polygyny because they'd rather share the healthiest male than have exclusive rights to the most faithful male. Nothing turns on a woman like a robust immune system. Repeat after me: In patriarchies with plenty of parasites, powerful parental providers get to be polygynous. Yay!

27.

Bimbos And Cuckolds: What Makes Us Jealous

I thought the swinger lifestyle would give me the love life of Don Juan. Instead it gave me the love life of Chief Inspector Clouseau. My girlfriend was Cato, randomly attacking me with emotional kung fu. Picture Jim Carrey in a porno movie. That was my life. A movie of my swinger years would be based on *Dumb and Dumber*, with me playing both parts. I had to weather the same indignities, the same physical pain, the same amount of ketchup sprayed in my face.

More than one-half of adulterous men describe their marriages as "happy." Men don't cheat because they're having marital problems. Supplemental sex is fun! Husbands are most likely to cheat between the ages of forty and sixty, when they are wealthiest. That's why the most virtuous men are those with no opportunities.

Most adulterous women say their marriage is "unhappy," and three-quarters say they are looking for a long-term commitment from their affair, which sounds to me like they are seeking to transition to a better mate.

A woman friend once told me a guy we knew was obviously sleeping around because he was insecure about how attractive he was. I stifled a laugh. I knew damn well why he was sleeping around: because it felt great. Women are the ones who sleep around because they feel bad about themselves. Men are more likely to sleep around when they feel great about themselves.

All the studies and surveys in the science journals can be summed up simply. Men are more likely to cheat because they are confident and horny. Women are more likely to cheat because they don't feel loved. Men want to be admired. Women want to be cherished. Women have sex to be loved. Men love to have sex.

But how do men and women feel about being cheated on? Psychologist David Buss pasted electrodes on men and women, asked them to imagine various treacheries involving their mates, and measured sweating, frowning, and heart palpitations.

Imagine your spouse having sex with the paperboy. Imagine discovering your spouse has been having secret picnics with a coworker for two years, yet they've never had sex. Imagine your spouse having a one-night stand, but never sees that person again. Imagine your spouse buying some expensive jewelry for a close friend you've never met—and you know your spouse hates shopping.

Buss explains the differences between men and women in clear lucid geek speak: "Skin conductance increased 1.4 microSiemens." "The electrode on the corrugator muscle of the brow . . . [showed] 7.75 microvolt units of contraction."

Those scientists. Always so sensationalistic. What he's trying to say is: men and women started sweating and frowning at different rates for different scenarios. Compare the body's reactions to the interviews, and you get a clear pattern.

Women feel more jealous over emotional attachment than sexual infidelity. Men feel more jealous over sexual infidelity than emotional attachment. Women worry about their mates having illicit sex to the extent it might lead to emotional bonds. Men worry about their mate's forming emotional bonds with men to the extent it might lead to illicit sex. The thought of their spouse's affair makes women more likely to experience humiliation and abandonment, and men more likely to feel humiliation and rage. The most extreme physiological reaction—when all the bouncing needles spiked terrifyingly high on the graph—was when men imagined their mate having hot sex with another man.

Why? A father can't be sure the kid is his. A mother can't be sure all her mate's resources are going to her kid.

When a baby comes out of your body, you can be sure it has your genes. When a baby comes out of somebody else's body, you can't be sure it has your genes. The wombless and bewombed have evolved different emotions when it comes to protecting their reproductive interests. Female jealousy guards resources. Male jealousy guards wombs.

These tendencies are only statistically, not universally, true. In any culture, you can find women who are more jealous over a one-night stand than secret picnics with secretaries, and males who are less threatened by sex with the paperboy as long as their wives love them. Eons of sexual selection have assured that the behavioral differences between men and women are analogous to differences in height. Some women are tall. Some men are short.

But the cross-cultural tendency toward taller men and shorter women is statistically overwhelming.

Many male chimps go nuts for the saggiest, most wrinkled female chimps. Age is cruel to *Homo sapiens* women because our brains are too big for easy births. This means pregnancy risks increase with age, which means our eyes have evolved to see beauty in female fertility, and youth is a sign of fertility. Since producing sperm is a lot less dangerous than bringing a human child to term, men remain fertile much longer, and our eyes have not evolved to see middle-aged men as unattractive. In fact we call them "distinguished," which means men are more likely to achieve distinction from the pack when they are older. The only things men "distinguish" themselves from are male losers, like book critics. It takes a lifetime for most men to win success, when suddenly their creaky bodies are in high demand and they start cheating as fast as they can before the prostate swells.

In fact, the less you are desired, the hornier you are. Sixteen-year-old boys are tormented by horniness, yet most women do not want them as husbands and fathers. Forty-year-old women are tormented by horniness, yet men are paying more attention to twenty-year-olds, many of whom haven't learned how to have orgasms yet. Nature fills us with desire when we are less desired.

Pleistocene men who preferred twenty-year-olds to forty-five-year-olds sired more children. Young women have more reproductive years ahead of them, and a higher chance of birthing healthy babies. Pleistocene women who preferred forty-five-year-olds to twenty-year-olds reared more children. A Pleistocene man who makes it to forty-five is more likely to have power and respect in the tribe than some young dork who might not make anything of himself. Many evolutionary biologists see the average age difference in marriage partners—very roughly four-and-a-half years—as a compromise between male and female interests. But many people range far outside this average. Most of these people are beautiful women and rich men.

The ethologist Karl Grammer studied a German dating service involving over 1,000 men and over 1,500 women and found that each increment in a male's income corresponded with a decrease in the age of the women sought. The more *deutsche marks*, the younger the *frauleins*.

The way many gays and lesbians conduct their love lives reveals what men and women really want. Lesbians I know have a joke: "First date, coffee. Second date, U-Haul." Commitment happens faster than men get to second base. Gay men have another joke: "First date, sex. Second date, learn each other's names." Another punchline is: "Second date? What's that?" Gay men I know have a standard retort when the stranger they just picked up in their car asks them their name: "Do you want to talk or have sex?" This usually causes them to zip it and unzip. Sex happens faster than they can drive home. I don't think this line would work on a woman.

Of course, many gay men are in committed relationships, and some lesbians are promiscuous. But the Kinsey Study of gay men in San Francisco conducted before the advent of AIDS showed that 75% of gay men had chalked up more than 100 partners, and 25% had more than 1,000. Yet most lesbians claimed fewer than ten partners in their lifetimes.

Heterosexual courtship and marriage represents a compromise between male and female desires. Women surrender when they have sex. Men surrender when they get married. Surrendering is a risk, and we only want to surrender to somebody we trust. Which is why lesbians are getting all the commitment and gay men are getting all the sex.

It turns out that, in the U.S.A., the best way to predict a man's wealth is to rate his wife's attractiveness, and the best way to predict a woman's attractiveness rating is her husband's wealth.

The richer men are, the more balls they have to request young and beautiful. The more beautiful women are, the more ovaries they have to request wealth and height. The rest of us watch entertainment about the rich and beautiful getting what they want. The TV show *Dallas* was very popular in societies like Pakistan, where marriages are arranged and women wear veils to protect men from their charms. Last I checked, *Baywatch* had a billion viewers, which means *Baywatch* earned as many converts in five years as Islam got in 1,000. Last time it showed, the art film *The Discreet Charm of the Bourgeoisie* had nine viewers. All of them live in Berkeley. When most people can't define half the words in your movie title, you know it's not meant for mainstream viewing. Compare the catchiness of *Baywatch* and the *Bible*, both of which are chock full of sex and status, you realize certain human preferences are universal.

Men are attracted to nubility and health. Women are attracted to nobility and wealth. Both want intelligence, kindness, and opulence. Both want a good sense of humor. They'll need it.

Women get older and steadily lower their mate standards. Men get richer and steadily raise their mate standards. We get married as our options narrow. If we can't get fertile bodies or fruitful resumes, we'll settle for amicable personality traits. Most of us marry our third or fourth choices.

"In every culture in the world. . .sex is seen as a service provided by females to males. In every culture, men are more violently jealous than women. All over the world, men are aroused more quickly than women, and men in every culture are more aroused by visual stimuli than women. The average husband is universally older than his wife, and the average man is universally more aggressive than the average woman. In every culture in the world, nubility is seen as a central attribute of female attractiveness for men, and high status is seen as a central attribute of male attractiveness for women."

—JAMES LETT, (1997) *Science, Reason and Anthropology: The Principles of Rational Inquiry*. Lanham, Maryland: Rowman & Littlefield.

Judging by the genetic rewards reaped by the dating games, Mother Nature favors us in this order: Most favored are high-status men. Second-most favored are beautiful, young women. Third-most favored are less attractive older women. Most lowly of all are low-status men—editors, for instance. (That's right, I'm talking to you, Samurai of the Red Pen.)

Eighty-percent of bull elephant seals never reproduce, yet one successful male can have over ninety offspring. Though 60% of female elephant seals are killed as youngsters, all of those who make it to adulthood get to have babies. The most successful females have ten offspring.

In virtually all species, Mother Nature has set things up so that most females pass on their genes, while most males die trying, and a very few elite males monopolize extra females. No matter how high the stakes get among females competing for pair-bonds, the stakes among males are much higher, which is why males are willing to die for sex.

More men than women die unmated. More men than women remarry after divorce and have more kids. More men than women die violently.

Youth passes, while status lasts—at least until younger apes take it from you. Young testosterone Turks are always out to knock the older leaders off their pedestals. Alpha men have allies and enemies, but few friends. Even though long childhoods require long pair-bonds which tone down the viciousness in males, sperm-makers of almost all species are designed to fight over wombs.

Age is not fair to women. Status is not fair to men. But all women get to be young, and most women pass on their genes. Few men get to be powerful, and many of them get to pass on extra genes, while many powerless men pass on none.

The drama in this dynamic doesn't just rage out there in the world. It rages inside you.

28.

Why You're Tormented

Maybe you're in a monogamous pair-bond. Yet, you still feel attracted to forbidden persons. Maybe you're single and sleep around. Yet, you still long for true love. Once we choose one reproductive strategy, why won't the other one go away? Why does being human have to be such a torment?

Our Big Problem is that hominid hierarchies were fluid across generations. Nobody likes to be the ape on the bottom, so tribal class structures underwent frequent upheaval. The children of low-status hominids could revolt and attain high-status positions. High-status people had babies with low-status people. I think you see the problem. These two opposing breeding strategies are not splitting into two separate species, *Homo promiscuous* and *Homo monogamous*. Sluts and prudes, interbreeding! This has caused the secret schizophrenic sexuality of every *Homo sapiens* you meet.

Yes, our ancestors had enough sex to mix up all the nice and naughty genes inside each of us. This means each of us is antagonistic toward the repressed side of ourselves, a dynamic that had kept many a therapist in business. Loyal wives are hostile toward the hussies who flirt with their husbands. Low-status concubines are hostile toward the goody-two-shoes who had high-status daddies and get high-status husbands. Yet, concubines want to be wives, and wives wish they could be a little wilder and get wild genes. Husbands agree with their wives that those loose wild women don't deserve respect, yet they also really want to have sex with them. And even the wild women won't have sex with them without some gesture of investment, which will really piss off the wife. I used to be one of those freewheeling bachelors who had disdain for the gentlemen who chain themselves to some bossy wife—*no woman will hold* me *down, man*—yet as I got grayer, I whimpered myself to sleep, dreaming of heirs and a cozy wife to take care of me.

Deep wishes are better dealt with when we can find an enemy who personifies them. Luckily there are always other *Homo sapiens* around.

Howard Bloom tells a great story in his *The Lucifer Principle: A Scientific Expedition into the Forces of History*.

Soon after Ronald Reagan was voted into his first presidential term, a group of Christian wives from Orange County, California suspected that secular humanism was teaching their children to be perverts. The women studied their children's grammar school textbooks under a microscope, and sure enough, the ladies found tiny X-rated pictures hidden inside the textbook illustrations. The crusade began. They made such a public stink, the grammar schools changed their textbook pictures for fear of alienating Christian parents.

One problem. The textbook illustrators had not hidden any erections or breasts in the minutiae of their drawings. The Christian wives of Orange County were looking at what amounted to Rorschach ink blot tests that revealed their own hidden fantasies. The Orange County goody-two-shoes had found their enemy, and the enemy was themselves. Inside every prude is an orgiast waiting to get out.

It's why happy housewives read dirty romance novels and happy husbands have the wandering eye problem. It's why studs and sluts are secretly lonely.

It's why danger is sexy. The evolution of sociality causes the evolution of sexual attraction to danger. Why? Kin try to control whom you mate with. Genes tell you to mix with foreigners. If your kin network disapproves of your lover, that's a sure sign that your lover has foreign genes. And there's nothing sexier, and more dangerous, than a stranger.

That's why "miscegenation"—a racist's word for interracial mating—is the hope for the human race. No matter how much we teach our children to hate the foreign race, we can't stop them from having sex with the foreign race. That's what members of the same species always want to do: boff their way to genetic diversity. Primates are always fornicating with the foreigners their fathers were fighting. Our great-great-grandchildren are destined to be beige.

Look at the history of population drift for the last few thousand years. Every generation is the mongrel mix of the people who were at war one hundred or ten or two generations ago. Lots of historians have wondered about the mysterious force for peace that has steadily changed us from tiny squabbling tribes of a few hundred people, to giant squabbling nations of hundreds of millions.

I can tell you exactly what this force for peace is. We *Homo sapiens* are even hornier than we are homicidal. The pattern of history when human tribes meet usually goes: war, rape, pillage, trade, intermarriage, mongrel babies.

I came of age under Reagan and Stallone. I spent my testosterone-fueled teenagerhood preparing for World War III. After the fall of the Berlin Wall, it took me three years to sleep with a Russian. Not long before, I was prepared to march to war against her brothers. But something about her dogmatic Socialist accent made my genitalia salute, and my decadent Western greed made her raise the Iron Curtain for a forbidden bad boy. We argued about ideology, called each other "commie slave" and "capitalist pig," and then had at each other like rabbits.

A whole lot of babies got conceived immediately after australopithecine mate fights. That's why we like violence and sex to go together in our entertainment, where we vicariously experience urges we're too secure and scared to pursue.

It was a high stakes game. Hominids who had risky sex with strangers passed on more genes than hominids who inbred with tribe-mates. But hominids who bred with respected neighbors were less often exiled or executed than promiscuous members of their community. As we survey our sexual landscape, we all weigh the tension between the risks required for genetic diversity and the calculation required for community support.

That's why we *Homo sapiens* are all a bunch of psychotically prudish sluts. Our hearts long for exclusive love, and our loins lust for chimp-style orgy. Plato's intuition about the charioteer of reason reining in the wild horses of passion was, neurologically, right on the money. We evolved neocortexes to inhibit instincts for long-term strategies in a social context, but the reptile and mammal parts of our brains still cry out for fulfillment. We keep our contradictory desires pitted against each other, weigh risks and consequences in our community, spasmodically act or make a sober choice, and then spend the rest of our lives fantasizing about the road not taken. Genes want all your breeding strategies primed to go, while you study the power relationships among your neighbors and give one strategy the go-ahead. Genes don't want you fulfilled. They want you to make and rear babies. A creature built to have contradicting desires is going to have a hard time fulfilling all of them.

But we don't want conflict! Organisms hate conflict! (Except for a few of my relatives, who live for it.)

This is one of the many examples of how competition is not about creatures, but about genes. Sometimes genes in different organisms make the organisms compete with each other. Sometimes competing genes in the same organism make the organism compete with itself. We are like big tanks that they drive, and half their conflicts go on inside the tank. Conflict we owe to the genes, whether it be external or internal.

Obviously, all your genes had better work together if they want to get their little deoxyribonucleic asses into the next generation, and it helps nobody if the pancreas is squabbling with the colon. (Though this was my Aunt Louise's precise problem.) Nevertheless, different parts of your brain sabotage each other. When we fall in love; when we force ourselves not to eat that donut; when we start falling asleep right when we need to concentrate; when we drink coffee to stop falling asleep and concentrate; when we lose our temper; when we conveniently "forget" to call our mother; when we train on the NordicTrack when we want to sleep in; when we say it's wrong to be attracted to our husband's brother, but our eyes keep looking at his butt. Different brain parts have different goals. In a brain your size, you're going to have a whole lot of complicated sub-goals, and brain mechanisms that specialize in pursuing them. All to pass on your genes. We humans can make anything complicated.

That's where "you" come in. The subjective self-conscious "you" (neocortex) evolved to work among your squabbling options in a social context—to make the best guess for attainment of friendship, status, good terms with neighbors, safe families, pair-bonds, and ass. Your job: build a working model for other brains, build a self-justifying model for your own brain, and start strategizing.

It is our very internal strife that leads to our amazing flexibility and adaptability. We humans have *more* instincts than do less flexible (and less neurotic) animals. Rattlesnakes are a bundle of efficient instincts, and they don't need therapy. They're not self-conscious, because they're not social, so they didn't evolve to make models of everybody's minds, including their own. Rational thought comes from compromise among competing instincts. Only a social animal can second-guess himself, doubt his impulses. If everything inside you went smoothly—mating, fighting, laying eggs, eating—you would have no internal conflict and need no neurotic neocortex.

Of course you're conflicted, you horny little monkey. As measured by surviving babies, the sins of the hypothalamus paid off as much as the civilized choices of the neocortex.

This drives us so crazy we could just die.

29.
Dying for Sex

Douglas Adams, in his *The Restaurant at the End of the Universe*, writes a scene set in the future where aliens have bred cows to not only talk, but to beg to be eaten. Before they prance into the oven, they present themselves to the dinner guests and invite them to poke their tender and juicy rumps. It's funny, because it seems ridiculous. You couldn't select for genes that make an animal want to be eaten. Could you?

The male black widow back-flips into the female fangs in the middle of copulation. The female black widow eats his butt while she engages in necrophilia with him.

Stupid? The male's suicide is a strategic move. Males who allow courtship to end in cannibalism pass on more genes than males who survive sex, because giving the female a full meal decreases her chance of mating again and introducing rival sperm. What a smart suicide!

He probably isn't calculated about it. Genes just make him stupid and impulsive. As to the universality of this strategy for male reproduction, I'll wait for all the facts to come in.

Moderate feminists can find little ideological support in the animal kingdom. In almost all species, males are more aggressive and dominant and insensitive, and females more interested in rearing young.

Radical feminists, however, can find plenty of support in the insect queendom. Female insects are often larger, more aggressive, and smarter than males. While engaged in coitus, the female preying mantis decapitates her lover and drinks his neck blood, which actually *improves* the headless male's performance. All sorts of metaphors can be derived from this, which I refuse to entertain here.

Courtship can get you killed. Many animals risk all for romance. A lightning bug's lantern flash of love, cast like a semaphore across the night, makes him easy prey for bats. The female mosquito's wail is music to the male's ears, yet grating to the ears of the giant whose blood she needs to feed her babies.

In the design of organisms, Mother Nature shows again and again that sex is more important than survival. If genes for risking your life for a brief moment of passion get you more surviving offspring than genes for staying alive, suicidal sexual behaviors will become prevalent in the population, even to the point of male spiders sacrificing their butts to the sexy female jaws of death. Freud would have a field day with the male spider.

Males are crazy because sperm are worthless. For males, showing off is more important than safety, because sex is more important than death. Every generation, some males will get extra wombs, but many more will die celibate. The competition among males is almost always more fierce, because the stakes for sperm-makers are higher.

Watch a male gazelle jump up and down to attract attention to himself when he sees the tiger. Won't that get him killed? Watch the peacock grow a giant entangling tail to make it easier for predators to nab him. Won't that get him killed? Watch the teenage boy race his hotrod down his residential street. Won't that get him killed? Watch twenty sea lions fight and bleed to hoard all the mates instead of divvying up the dates democratically. Won't that get them killed?

Survival is secondary. Sex is all. Your urge to survive was designed in service to your urge to reproduce. Luckily we have a neocortex, which is in charge of storing and passing information, so humans live far beyond their reproductive years in order to pass wisdom on to offspring. This makes bull elephant men more safety-conscious than bull elephant seals.

But the population geneticist Alan Rogers studied the insurance statistics and calculated that young men should severely discount the future, then steadily worry more about their future as they get older. If you're a young sperm-maker, you have the urge to take big risks. If you have a womb, young males who take risks seem insane. But the sanest way for a young sperm-maker to win the competition for wombs is to display his insanity to other sperm-makers. Virility *is* insanity. Testosterone drives animals to take risks, because sperm-makers play for higher stakes: lots of offspring, or no offspring at all.

Not only does this explain why one man is murderously jealous when somebody sleeps with his wife, it explains when another man is perfectly fine with somebody sleeping with his wife.

30.

When Your Wife Sleeps with Your Brother, and You're Okay with That

Polyandry is the marrying of one woman to two or more husbands. In a world dominated by polygyny, where men marry several women, this arrangement is a refreshing exception. It's especially strange when you consider that polyandrous cultures are patriarchal. The men are arranging for females to be double-diddled! The two husbands who share a wife are almost always brothers. Less than 1% of cultures allow a woman to marry two brothers, and they all have something in common: not enough territory.

Walk innocently across your neighbor's front lawn, and you will discover that *Homo sapiens* is a territorial animal. Mark his lawn with some harmless urine, and you will witness a passionate territorial reaction. *Homo sapiens* offspring like to expand into new territories

and create new families. Thus suburban sprawl. When males of territorial species can't secure any territory, females won't mate with
them. What happens when a whole tribe of *Homo sapiens* males run
out of territory into which to expand?

Most polyandrous societies are in isolated pockets of southern
Asia. We think of Tibet and think of spiritual satori. We should also
think of women with two husbands. I suspect this is why my girlfriend is so entranced by Tibet's version of enlightenment.

Then there are the Nair people, who inhabit India's Malabar
Coast, squeezed into small areas by dominant Brahmin. Many of
their women are kidnapped for the foreign sex trade, so women are
a minority there. There are the Japanese tribes in the high
Himalayas—the Sherpa, Bhutia, Lepcha. Also the Khasas of the
North-East, Todas of Tamil Nadu, the Nayars of Kerala. In all these
cultures, two brothers pass one wife back and forth between beds.

It's hard for men to stake expansive claims atop mountains, surrounded by mountains or oceans, or blocked off by overpowering
enemies who let you live on the marginalized lands that aren't worth
fighting for. When the land is barely fertile, sometimes it takes the
work of two men to support one woman and her children.

But male instincts are constructed to preserve family genes.
You don't want to share your wife with just anyone. When there's
not enough land to divvy up between brothers, two brothers will
work the same land and tend the same woman. I wish polyandry
were an arrangement made by Kandyan feminists of Sri Lanka, but
it ain't. Polyandry is a contract between two brothers to preserve
the family estate.

Even in polyandrous societies, men control women. The
women are forced into situations where, while one husband is
working the farm to feed her children, the other is massaging her

feet or satisfying her sexually. The husbands work in shifts, switching back and forth as a tag-team. No wonder Sri Lankan women are reluctant to be liberated.

Imagine you're a Sri Lankan parent with your little spot of crappy land. You have two sons. Should you split up the land so both your sons are half as wealthy as you? If you just give all the land to the older son, that means the younger one will starve, die celibate, or volunteer to be the elder's slave. (As the oldest son of a big family, I've always been a big fan of primogeniture.) Why waste calories on a second son who will never grow up to own territory and give you grandchildren?

To prevent dilution of wealth, the quantity strategy is foregone for the ultimate quality strategy: invest all family sperm and wealth in one womb to produce one high-status child. One grandchild with extra dads is better than many grandchildren of one dad. In cultures with no territory left to conquer, brothers all mate with one female and each raises the offspring as his own.

Polyandry prevents war. Population growth must be restricted, or famine will ensue. Men will start wars to prevent other men from having sex with their wives, yet brothers will share wives to prevent war. Our emotions usually provoke us to do what is best for our genes.

We're not the only territorial species whose behavior illustrates how the size of the male's territory determines the number of mates.

The male wattled jacana birds are seduced by deadbeat moms and abandoned to raise the chicks as single-parent dads. Often, many of the offspring are not even theirs. The scoundrelettes run around copulating an average of sixty-five times per brood, right in front of the male brooding over her eggs.

This startled biologists. How do we account for this sex-role reversal?

The answer? Limited territory for a territorial bird.

In highly competitive, heavily populated habitats with limited room for nests, many males must die bachelors. Jacanas evolved in limited-range territories. Males are lucky to inseminate any females at all, so polyandry became the norm. The best strategy for a male jacana is to mix his sperm in the womb with other sperm and hope for the best, even to the point of raising the chicks in case that they are his. Funny how when females control the sex, males turn into mensches.

Tasmanian hens are not exactly hotties. They look like turkeys. Yet some of them manage to keep two husbands handy. Why not? The average number of offspring for a monogamous hen is six-and-a-half. The average number for a polyandrous hen is nine-and-a-half.

Why do the husbands put up with it? Half of nine-and-a-half offspring is not as good as all of six-and-a-half. It only comes out to an average four-and-three-quarters offspring per male.

The answer? Only brothers share a wife. Since brothers share half their genes, they do their genes good sharing a hen. That way, each brother's genes are represented in an average of seven-and-a-quarter offspring, which is better than six-and-a-half.

So the old saw is true: A hen in one hand is better than six-and-a-half in the other. Or something.

How about actual turkeys? Alan H. Krakauer, a graduate student at U.C. Berkeley, found that turkey brothers will cooperate to get their biggest brother laid. Who would have guessed a turkey would make such a great wing man? While the dominant brother does the usual—flashes his colors, struts, and thrums his air sac—his brothers will flash their colors, too, but without the thrumming and strutting, sort of like Ricky Martin's backup dancers. They also face outward to ward off any interlopers who might try to throw the bro off his game. Krakauer studied the DNA of fifty-one males, seventy-five females, and 325 offspring and found that altruistic celibate brothers passed on extra genes. How? Because for every baby sired by a solitary male, dominant males with a posse of supporting brothers sired seven. The altruistic celibates were passing on more genes through their dominant brother than each could alone.

We easily forget that it's not the number of direct offspring that matters, but the percentage of genes passed on. If you can pass on more of your genes by sharing a wife with your brother, you'll evolve to be turned on by your brother diddling your wife. If you have territory to expand into and extra females to win, you'd rather kill your brother than let him diddle your wife.

I nearly killed my brother over a piece of birthday cake once; he'd better not even *look* at my girlfriend. But if our family didn't have any territory, our parents would be saying the same thing about my girlfriend that they said about my birthday cake: "Share with your little brother!" He'd barge into my bedroom and whine, "No fair! I want some!"

Eskimos don't possess the most fertile land in the world. Men sometimes share wives. But co-husbands keep murdering each other. Why can't Eskimos run a decent polyandrous society? Because Eskimo men share wives with non-kin. We can see how the differential survival of genes constructs emotions and predicts behavior. When the right percentage of a married male's genes is passed on, there is no murderous jealousy. When a small percentage of a married male's genes is passed on, there is murderous jealousy.

Male humans kill each other for pride, but male lions kill each other for prides. Yet, the best way to control a pride of lionesses is for some male lions to team up to fight off other males. How do lions agree to share a female? Coalitions are almost always formed among lions that grew up in the same litter: brothers, half-brothers, an occasional cousin, in rare cases one stranger. The success of this strategy has created selection pressure for lionesses to give birth to several sons at once, so they can grow to team up and control prides together.

Again and again in evolutionary biology, we see how animal behavior is elucidated by gene equations. Set up the parameters, run your equation through the computer, predict the behavior. Whatever works out best for genes ends up constructing our emotions. Evolutionary biologists already have gene equations that predict various forms of cooperation, competition, self-sacrifice, family love, and hostility.

Across the world, men with big territories or high prestige get extra wives, if they're lucky, and men with little territories get half a wife, if they're lucky. Dominant males didn't start hoarding hundreds of wives until the invention of agriculture. Among hunter-gatherers, a chieftain usually maintains five wives, tops.

So here's how it divvies up: Where there is lots of vegetable food, there are men with multiple wives. Where there is little vegetable food, there are women with multiple husbands.

I have mixed feelings reporting these facts, because now men are going to run for the vegetables, and women will sprint for the limited territory, and everybody will arrive in their paradise and meet nobody from the opposite sex.

If you want to sleep with your husband's brother, you have to live in an enclosed area with not enough food and territory to go around. You know how men are about food and territory. His family will beg you to double-diddle.

Also, ladies, to get extra men working to support you, you

don't need the perfect body. You just need to move the body you got to the culture where it's most appreciated.

31.

Broad Hips, Big Butts; Broad Shoulders, Big Diction

The Hadza men of Tanzania, who, like our ancestors, live in a mixed savanna and woodland habitat, love the fat women. The fatter the better. In societies where women's work is energetically expensive, a woman's girth is a sign that she is a good gatherer and so popular among women she doesn't have to work too hard. Fatness is also a sign of early puberty, late menopause, and regular ovulations. Yum-yum. Let's not even talk about lactation capacities. You have to have status to maintain all that fat.

Parisian men who, unlike our ancestors, live in a city of sofas and gooey pastries on every corner, love the thin women. The thinner the better. In societies where fried food is everywhere and aortas look like the insides of a mayonnaise jar, thin women live longer; tend to have more wealth and more time to exercise. Maintaining a low-fat diet is actually expensive in industrialized countries, whereas less wealthy people have access mostly to high-fat food. You have to have status to stay so skinny.

Two researchers named Stunkard and Sobal looked at 144 studies of the relation between wealth and weight and found two strong correlations going in opposite directions on the graph. In Western countries, the lower the average woman's weight, the higher her status. In societies with food scarcities, the higher the average woman's weight, the higher her status.

To prepare for weddings in Beverly Hills, brides exile themselves to "fat farms" or join Weight Watchers to slim down for the dress. Among the Annang of Nigeria, brides are secluded in "fattening rooms" to plump them up for sex. Their personal trainers put them on a strict regimen. No exercise allowed. Non-stop gorging is enforced. When the Annang girls emerge plump enough to ovulate and mate, other girls look upon their temporary rotundity with envy.

In well-fed cultures, thin women are preferred, because it's harder to be thin. In poorly-fed cultures, fat women are preferred, because it's harder to be fat. No matter where you go, men prefer the shape that's hardest to be.

Most societies throughout history have preferred the plump women. That's because most societies throughout history have sucked. According to historian Roberta · Seid, once our society became overfed, that thinness became a "preference" at the turn of the century, a "prejudice" during the 1950's, a "myth" in the 1960's, an "obsession" in the 1970's, and a "religion" in the 1980's. Peruse the nearest issue of "*Prettier Than You Magazine*," and you'll see what I mean. The richer we get, the thinner we like our women. Do you have any idea how difficult it is to look like a concentration camp victim in Manhattan? Look at that perfume billboard: dark circles under her eyes, ribs poking through, no breasts, no hips, sullen, bored pout—talk about sexy!

When peasants worked in fields and aristocrats sat in castles, pale skin was considered beautiful among Caucasians. When the industrial revolution required laborers to work indoors, and only the wealthy could afford vacations to exotic locales, a strong tan was considered beautiful among Caucasians. Within a generation of any nation being conquered, the conquered learn to find their conquerors more attractive. That's because conquerors have more prestige.

Cross-cultural variability in beauty tastes reveals one constant: prestige is beautiful. Symbols of status change. Attraction to status does not, even if rich teens decide the true mark of status is connection with the gritty streets. Third-world men like 'em fat and fair. Industrialized men like 'em thin and tanned. Whatever symbolizes high status, we try to screw it.

But there is one standard of female beauty that is set in stone—actually, bone. And fat. It is shared by virtually all cultures and allows almost no variability. All men everywhere like the same waist-to-hip ratio: .70, meaning the waist is exactly 70% the size of the hips.

The .70 waist-to-hip ratio is so exacting, it holds across all body types. Those Hadza Tasmanian devil-men like them plump and juicy at .70. Rural Jamaicans like that hookah-shape .70, mon. Ancient "Venus" figurines found in sites from Europe to Asia are enormously fat, and most maintain the golden ratio of fecundity: .70. If the prehistoric sculptors were men, it looks like they preferred the universal waist-to-hip ratio, but they weren't sticklers for the universal fact that women have heads. Women on the dating scene have also made this observation.

Look at all the Miss Americas from 1920 through the 1980s. Some of them are voluptuous. Some of them are svelte. All eighty of them show waist-to-hip ratios between .69 and .72. How about classic beauties? Sophia Loren, Audrey Hepburn, and Marilyn Monroe all had .70 waist-to-hip ratios—at least during times when we paid attention to them. What about the extremes like teeny Twiggy and amazon Elle McPherson? In their heyday Twiggy was a .73 and Elle was a .69. Even tiny Kate Moss was right on the money, .70.

Studies of the history of painting and sculpture in a variety of cultures in Egypt, Africa, India and Greece over the last 500 years reveal that weights can range up and down, but waist-to-hip ratios remain the same. The same was demonstrated by a detached scientific scrutiny of *Playboy* centerfolds, which for some reason didn't need to be funded.

There is one known exception: The isolated Matsigenka of southeast Peru seem to prefer women with high waist-to-hip ratios. They like 'em tubular. One man described a silhouette with a .70 waist-to-hip as looking like she had diarrhea.

Eskimo women have body fat that is more evenly distributed all over their bodies for better insulation, so their waist-to-hip ratio is less pronounced.

American men shown pictures of rainforest Yanomamo women picked the same most attractive women as the Yanomamo tribesmen. American and Asian men agreed separately on the most desirable American and Asian women. South African and American men agreed on which South African and American women they wanted to do. The Chinese, Indian, and English men all agreed on the same hotties. Female beauty always means signs of health and fertility. Men want them ripe.

Fashions throughout European history show men padding shoulders and crotches, and women doing crazy things with corsets, bodices, crinolines, and bustles. Women have even removed ribs in their effort to get closer to that exact .70 symbol of fertility. A waist is a terrible thing to mind.

Most healthy pre-menopausal women range between .67 and .80, while most men who are not obese have waist-to-hip ratios of .85 to .95. That's a big difference. It's hard to maintain a waist. So why do women have to do all the waist-maintaining?

We are the only species that has a waist. Prepubescent girls don't have waists. Post-menopausal women don't have waists. Women evolved waists to show they can birth babies with big heads. Men evolved attraction to waists, because it makes hips look bigger, and big hips means big-brain-birthing talents. It is in women's interests to store fat on their butts and thighs to exaggerate hip size. Thighs account for one-quarter of a woman's weight. Aren't you women lucky!

We all are. We owe human evolution to women's waists. Hominid women's hips evolved to get wider and wider until they reached the absolute limit past which they could not walk. If you're a nomadic species, you have to walk. Now big-brained babies had to be birthed earlier and earlier, which means much of the brain-building went on not inside the womb, but outside in the community, which means we became a culturally malleable animal, which made us geniuses.

Yet hips became like a peacock's tail: the other sex likes it, so it keeps evolving whether it's practical or not. Hips could not get any wider, so waists got slimmer. Women evolved slim waists to fake out men. Men think the hips are big, but actually the waist is small. Yet still the competition for men continued. So, fertile women evolved to keep fat away from their bellies and put it all on their hips and breasts. When you're a sex which has to compete for mates, you can't announce too much fertility.

Apes are born with huge brains, but they are only half as big as they will grow after birth. Humans are exceptional. We are born with brains that are only one-third grown. Yet a human baby's brain is completely out of proportion to the rest of the body. The head is so heavy the newborn can't lift it off the ground. The little creature won't even be able to walk for ten months to a year. That long infancy and endless teenagerhood is a heavy price to pay for such a big brain.

Maybe we should use them. I have scientific proof that, when it comes to criticizing our reflections in the mirror, we should all give ourselves a break. Especially you women. Okay, so maybe when you bend over at the beach, people think there's an eclipse. So what? Judging by the following scientific study, your ass is not all it's cracked up to be.

American men and women were shown illustrations of men and women. All the cartoons looked the same, except they ranged from fat to slim. Women were asked which cartoon guy was the most attractive. They mostly picked the guy with the moderate waist-to-shoulder ratio. More women picked the slightly chubby guy than the super he-man guy.

Then they asked the women to choose which cartoon gal they thought men found most attractive. Most women chose the super-slim cartoon.

Then they asked men which cartoon gal they found most attractive. Though men picked within a narrower range than women, almost all the men picked the moderately slim but still buxom cartoon. Very few picked the super-slim cartoon.

Then they asked men to pick which cartoon guy they thought women found most attractive. Most men picked the he-man guy.

Both men and women overestimate what the other sex wants. Women think men like the ultra-skinny women, when most American men like the moderately slim but full-figured woman. Men think women like the bodybuilder types, but women really like the solid types, and some women even like the chubbier ones best.

In other words, you look sexier than you think you do.

Remember Marilyn Monroe was a size 16, but a perfect .70, and she is responsible for a half-century of male orgasms.

But it still seems unfair. Some women picked the chubbier guy. How come American men don't like chubby women? Well, they do, but only to the extent the waist-to-hip ratio is more important than signs of skinny status. The researchers took aside the men who liked the skinny cartoon gal. They showed those men a fat cartoon woman with a .70 waist-to-hip ratio and a thin woman with a higher waist-to-hip ratio. Most of those men preferred the fat woman with the magical hourglass .70. Signs of status are variable. The waist-to-hip ratio is eternal.

But forget your butts and guts. I'll tell you what really gets you laid: bullshit. If you can't talk up a storm, you'll die celibate. Here's my scientific proof:

You know about 60,000 words. You only use 4000 of them regularly. The other 56,000 account for 2% of your speaking.

Pick a word from that extra 56,000. You use it about once every million words you speak. A million words is about twenty times the number of words in this book. To function socially in the world, you need fewer than 1,000 words. Out of your bloated vocabulary of 60,000 words, one hundred words account for 60% of your conversation. So why did you memorize 60,000 words?

You big show off! Whom are you trying to impress?

Mates.

And since you are from a tribal, gossipy species, that means you better impress everyone if you want to impress your mate. The hugest bulk of human vocabulary is purely ornamental. There is no point in saying you want to copulate, mate, screw, ball, mount, make love, ravish, seduce, despoil, or deflower when a perfectly serviceable word like boink will do. Your vocabulary is a peacock's big tail.

Vocabulary varies greatly among people, showing vocabulary is a sexually selected trait. It's also plenty wasteful, like all sexy traits should be. Children must learn about fifteen words a day for eighteen years before they get anywhere near their 60,000. This is a tremendous waste of brain power that could be spent on something useful like learning how to grow their own food or amortize their parents' mortgage. But no, the little punks would rather talk. They'll need to if they want to out-flirt their competitors.

Guys, I don't care if it does work for the gibbon, yelling "woo" when you see a fertile rump won't get you sex. We need wit to woo. Our peacock tails are human tales. They display the health of our sexiest organ—how clever, colorful, and creative it is. Obscenely huge vocabularies are display traits that evolved because they got our ancestors sex. Which is why I sesquipedalianize my antidisestablishmentarianism so supercallifragilisticexpialidociously.

Hey, I think I just coined my new pick-up line.

Wait, I've got an even better pick-up line.

32.

Why Your Penis Is Easy to Find

Let's start off with a scientific fact: I have a humongous penis.
Compared to an ape, anyway. Compared to most apes, even the
most poorly endowed male *Homo sapiens* is super-hung.

The fully erect penis of the "Testicle King" chimp is (snicker)
three inches. The fully erect penis on an orangutan is (chuckle)
one-and-a-half inches. The fully erect penis on the tough-guy
gorilla is (nyah-ha!) one-and-a-quarter inches. When these guys'
dongs aren't erect, you can't even see them.

The stiff *Homo sapiens* schlong is on average five inches long,
and it's clearly visible when we aren't even using it. Some biologists believe we walk upright to show it off.

Let's consult the insight of Andrea Dworkin:

"The penis must embody the violence of the male in order for him to be male. Violence is male; the male is the penis; violence is the penis or the sperm ejaculated from it. What the penis can do it must do forcibly for a man to be man."

—ANDREA DWORKIN, (1981) *Pornography: Men Possessing Women*

I can't help feeling that somewhere in here I'm being called a dick. What these ultra-feminists don't understand is that you can't just go around slandering the penis. This symbol of male power is also the most delicate body part we men have. The pathology that results from this Penis Paradox is the cornerstone upon which civilization was built. How would you like it if some civilization used your clitoris as a cornerstone? Imagine if the Washington Monument looked like a moist engorged clitoris. Maybe then women would feel some inkling of our pressure to perform. The Leaning Tower of Pisa gives me the creeps. They should have called it The Almost-Drooping Tower of Pisa. That's why the Italians lost the war.

For men's obsession with their own penises, women have their own selves to blame.

Here's my scientific proof: remember when we distinguished traits designed by natural selection (to solve problems in nature) from traits designed by sexual selection (to solve problems with the opposite sex)?

Dicks don't solve problems in nature. Nobody ever lassoed a wildebeest with his penis. As far as natural selection is concerned, penises have one purpose: shoot sperm. The energy spent to build a gorilla's stubby, skinny pud is all natural selection is willing to give it.

Natural selection hones all attributes down to their minimalist, most efficient design, and gives every organism in the species the same design. The pinky-sized gorilla penis is a perfect specimen of a trait created by natural selection.

Homo sapiens penises have all the attributes of something designed by sexual selection: Penises are "age-specific," meaning they reach full size only after puberty. Penises are "courtship-specific," meaning they bloat to display size only at times of courtship. Penises look different on different men. When it's hard, it's not hard to find. Like peacock tails, penises evince strong reactions in females, either of revulsion, excitement, or withering indifference. All this tells us the human penis was designed by female choice.

Oversized schlongs, to natural selection, have no point. Whenever you see something pointless on a male animal, you can bet it's there by female choice. Penises, like all sexually selected traits, are designed to show off how much energy they can waste.

Other primates get to have bones in their boners. When a male chimp notices a female in estrus, his pencil-thin prick snaps into position like something out of a *Penthouse* cartoon. Almost all the moveable parts in your body require bones. Even something as lightweight as your ear requires stiff cartilage to hold it up.

Yet selection by females has bred *Homo sapiens* males to have boneless boners. The human penis is an inflatable blood balloon. No wonder it looks kind of funny. To lift a slab of flesh and hold it aloft without a bone requires some serious hydraulics. The *Homo sapiens* male wastes no time borrowing energy from his immune system to raise his testosterone (dick fuel), thus raising his chances of disease. This is like cutting off supplies to the microscopic troops at the front so you can engorge some kingly ornament with an energy feast. Yet another way that males risk death for sex.

But death does not scare men as much as impotence. Men are insecure about their penises because of an instinctive understanding that, like peacock's tails, erections are the most honest indicator of how healthy we are. Any number of small things can go wrong, and erections won't work. I won't get into it here, because I'm afraid I'll jinx myself.

It's the same with bower bird bowers or toucan tails or gibbon hoots, or any other display of male virility. One microscopic virus, one teeny cancerous mutation, an inability to find good nutrition, and females can see it in the "primary fitness indicator," whether it be a brain, bower, or boner. A peacock displaying his flawless tail is saying, "Look how much energy I can waste on my perfectly symmetrical tail! No parasites! No bad genetic mutations! C'mon, baby, let's do it like they do on the *Discovery Channel!*"

The more hominid females chose males based on pointless penis feats, the more the penis evolved to show off the difficulty of its stunts. "Now," announces the show-off penis, "I will perform an upright erection without a bone, lifting ten times my weight, borrowing half the brain's blood!"

Females say "oooo," collect the big-penis genes, and next generation, the dick has to raise the bar once again. A few million years of this, you end up with your ridiculously oversized boneless boner.

Males of species with lots of display strutting often don't have much in the way of ornaments on their genitals. Egrets leap and cavort around, and you can't even see their penises.

Males of a species with fancy ornaments on their genitals often have less display strutting. Mandrill monkeys with psychedelic scrotums have nothing to prove. They know they're cool.

Males of most species get either big dances or big dicks. Do some anthropological research at your local dance club, and you'll notice most male *Homo sapiens* don't dance very well. My groovin' booty bumps rarely have the seductive effect I intend.

I think this trade-off between aggressive behavior and large penises has something to do with how some men drive. For instance, I drive my small stubby white car quite calmly.

Gorilla males beat their chests. Chimp males do charging displays. Great white egrets dance. We humans have titanic penises. And those who don't, drive SUVs.

If we have women to blame for our big balls, we have women to thank for our giant penises. Females decided to breed males for larger and more gravity-defying penises. Thus, men's obsession with their dicks is all women's fault. I rest my case.

I've got more bad news for the married. Monogamous primate penises tend to be tiny. The faithful owl monkey male might as well not even have a penis, it's so dinky. Promiscuous primate penises tend to be huge, because of competition to deliver sperm closer to the target. Next time your wife claims she's faithful, point to your penis and say, "Oh yeah? Then how come my dick is so big?" Next time your husband swears he was out with the boys, say, "Prove it! Show me your tiny owl monkey penis!"

If you want to measure the significance of female choice to our evolution, the penis is the perfect yardstick. The *Homo sapiens* prick was engineered, designed, and enlarged by female decisions, the design passed down through generations of women, each molding the penis to her specifications, each coming up with the many different designs we can see modeled on many different men. The soft, elegant, vulnerable penis is a feminine sculpture. That's why we're protective of them.

Once hominid men and women began choosing each other's erogenous zones as signs of reproductive fitness, things got out of hand. To attract men, women evolved pointlessly perky breasts that actually make it *harder* to nurse infants. Infants and adult men compete over the same female breast. Infants want them small and efficient squirters of milk. Men want them over-bloated with fat so they only *seem* like efficient squirters of milk. Women's breasts range widely in size and shape, they waste a lot of energy, and they are inconvenient: perfect evidence that they evolved through male choice.

Our hands do more than fashion tools and civilizations. They fashion our physical forms. A man's hands on a woman's body are, in a sense, sculpting her. His choices bred her to have rounded breasts and an hourglass shape, both exaggerated displays of baby-making talents that serve no practical purpose except to attract mates.

Some evolutionary biologists have come up with a supplemental penis theory. It's possible that penis size was a sign of status among early hominid hunters. Often "sexually dimorphic" traits evolve because of their effect on same-sex members of the species. Vervet monkeys, when threatened, posture, make mean faces, and sprout erections from their red, white, and blue genitalia.

Dr. R.H. Stubbs, a professional penis-lengthener who is one of my heroes in the realm of overcoming name disability, noted that a majority of men who apply for penis enlargement cite locker room embarrassment, yet only a third cite bedroom embarrassment. This may not be as quirky as it sounds. Certainly big muscles are more important to men than to women. That's because muscles served more to intimidate men than attract women. If penis size conferred status among hominid males, and status led to more surviving offspring, then male choice might also have had a hand in sculpting the penis.

Religious leaders tell us our bodies were fashioned by the

hand of God, but biology tells us our penises *might* have been fashioned by the hand of a certain kind of man.

33.

Two Genes for Two Types of Gay Guys

Homosexuality runs in families. Gay men have more gay brothers. Lesbian women have more lesbian sisters. Is it environmental or genetic?

A team of five geneticists took a survey and found that the chances that anyone's brother is gay are 2%.

Then they studied seventy-six gay men and found that about 14% of their brothers were gay, about 7% of the male cousins on their mothers' side were gay, and about 7% of their mothers' brothers were gay.

Yet the incidence of homosexuality among all other male relatives was about 2%, just like it is for the rest of the population.

Then they took a survey and found that the chances that anyone's sister is a lesbian are 1%.

Among these same seventy-six gay men, about 5% of their sisters were lesbians. They also found that about 5% of the brothers of lesbians were gay.

Yet the incidence of homosexuality of all other female relatives was about 1%, just like the rest of the population.

If homosexuality was caused by how they were raised, why weren't there more homosexuals among the dads' relatives? Like male baldness, male homosexuality seems to be passed down mostly along the maternal line.

Are all these statistical analyses boring you? I'm sorry. I'm getting bored myself, considering I haven't typed the word *penis* in a whole page. Science is hard. Cheap dick jokes are not so hard.

Yet there is something curious in the numbers. You'll notice the frequency of gays among mom's brothers and male cousins on mom's side is only half that of brothers. If gayness was inherited from one gene, homosexuality among mom's brothers and male cousins should be higher, between three-quarters to equal that of brothers.

Also, the rate of gay males among all non-maternal relatives was 2%, while the rate of lesbians was 1%. Among these seventy-six gay men, the rate of lesbian sisters was only half that of gay male cousins on mom's side, and only a third as much as gay brothers.

By now I'm sure you've solved these hilarious equations in your head. The only way the researchers could make the numbers work was to hypothesize *two types of homosexuality*, one type that was only male and came from the mother, and one type that was either male or female and could come from either parent.

Time for a new experiment. They looked at thirty-eight families that had two homosexual brothers. They made a prediction. If there are two genes for homosexuality, in this set they should see higher rates of homosexuality in the gay man's mother's relatives, closer to three-quarters of that found in brothers, whereas rates of homosexuality in the father's relatives should stay the same.

They ran the survey. The prediction was almost exact. Mom's gay brothers and male cousins on mom's side rose from fifty to seventy-five percent. The rates of homosexuality among the father's relatives remained unchanged.

There is not a gay gene. There are *two* gay genes in males, on different parts of the genome, each favored by natural selection as reproductive strategies. Homo *Homo sapiens* males evolved not once but twice.

Why?

Hang on, science boy. There's still more boring lab work to do. Unsheathe your electron microscope and turn on the centrifuge. Don the cool orange goggles.

Can we link these surveys to specific genes? The researchers looked at DNA from forty pairs of homosexual brothers, and found 82.5% of them had the now legendary Xq28 on the X-chromosome inherited from their mothers. The chances of this occurring by coincidence are less than one in one hundred. Though this result was not confirmed by a later experiment, it certainly got attention.

Scientists may have isolated a gay gene. The trick is not to ostracize it.

So does Xq28 *cause* you to be gay? Not exactly, because genes express themselves in cooperation with other genes though environmental triggers. But if a man has the Xq28 gene, the chances that he is gay are higher.

Hey, gay men. Next time you go clubbing, scan the room. Can you see two different types of gay guys?

Though we lab technicians will give you scientific confirmation for only two, homophiles in the field report there are a lot more. Amateur anthropologists have captured, marked, and set free enough specimens to organize a whole periodic table: bois, boyz, drag kings, gender outlaws, m2fs, pansexuals, stone butches, rainbow queers, radical fairies, shemales, ladyboys, leatherlads, science boys. I wish these terms had a little more scientific respectability— something Latin perhaps—but this is what happens when amateur studiers of the *Homo* genus do all the hands-on field research. Despite their lack of grants, these renegade researchers found some mysterious means of motivation. They have inexhaustibly collected enough fluid samples to suggest that human sexual behaviors vary along a diverse and unpredictable range.

A gene for homosexuality could only have secured so large a role in the human family if it somehow conferred tremendous reproductive power to nieces and nephews—so tremendous, in fact, that it would have offset the reproductive disadvantage of not directly procreating. In other words, gay genes can only copy themselves through family values. And that's assuming homosexuals would have had no children, which is not a sound assumption. Were homosexual women and men vital providers to their kin in Pleistocene communities?

Nobody has convincingly established that modern homosexual aunts and uncles invest more resources in their nieces and nephews than heterosexual aunts and uncles. But should we infer that this must have been so in the ancestral past of all species with homosexuals among them?

There's only one place to look: gay aunts and uncles in other species.

34.
Gay Animal Parents

Has the whole world turned gay? Birds and bees, butterflies and beetles, cockroaches and crickets, dolphins and deer, gorillas and geese, octopi and orcas, pigeons and porcupines, whales and warthogs. Girly-boy guinea pigs. Butch lesbian penguins that beat up males. Fruity fruit bats. Bear bears. Not to mention those all-male orgiasts, the (ahem) bighorn rams. These guys really go at it, in big beastly groups without a female in sight. Talk about a wild kingdom. Next time somebody tells you homosexuality is unnatural, point him to nature.

A straight male ostrich courts a female with a restrained display and a romantic song. But the fabulous display of ostriches that court fellow males steals the show. Gay ostriches charge their objects of affection at 30 MPH, skid to a stop just before collision, pirouette, fluff their feathers, and twist their necks into a corkscrew. They don't even bother with the song. Two percent of male ostriches do this, and the males they court aren't always obviously gay, though—who knows?—maybe the court-ers have some kind of gaydar we don't have.

There is even a species that has never been observed to mate heterosexually. Its members have only been observed to mate homosexually. The species is called (I swear) the black-rumped flameback. To spare it all the jokes, I'd call it by its more general name if it wasn't "woodpecker." Since the species keeps reproducing, some deviant heterosexual flamebacks must be secretly mating somewhere.

And homos make good parents.

Male pink flamingoes have sex, build nests, and rear foster chicks together. They don't seem to mind being pink.

Female grizzlies form lifelong pair-bonds, raise cubs together, and even put off hibernation to share more time together, like dorm girls staying up late to talk.

Straight bottlenose dolphins don't form lifelong pair-bonds. Only gay bottlenose dolphins form lifelong pair-bonds. Some bottlenose dolphins are exclusively gay. This is an aberration against nature, since most bottlenose dolphins are bisexual. Their brains are also bigger than ours.

The animal most genetically similar to humans is the bonobo chimp. Every single bonobo is bi. They also cuddle more than we do, fight less, are feminist, and get a lot more sex.

Humans may isolate the gay gene, but we can't seem to exclude it. There it is, snuggled cozily inside our genome, as if it had some hand in assuring our species' survival. Isn't a gene's success determined by how many copies of itself it produces in offspring? How would evolution select for sex that doesn't even produce offspring? It seems like a big mystery until you look at a black swan's gay uncle.

Gay black swans form permanent pair-bonds, and since they are both males, they can defend territories much larger than those of straight couples. The homosexual swans adopt or kidnap eggs, raise chicks, and, on average, raise *twice* as many offspring to breeding age as straight couples.

If you are straight, and your sibling is gay, there's a strong chance you carry recessive gay genes. You can pass on your genes by helping one of your offspring to survive, or you can pass on even more genes by helping three nieces or nephews to survive. If gay swans get their eggs from siblings often enough, and raise nieces and nephews at double the rate that straight siblings can raise their own kids, simple mathematics tells us gay genes could be favored in the population.

Lesbian couplings in ring-billed gulls and California gulls improve gene reproduction as well. To raise gull chicks, you need a two-parent family. One earns the bacon; the other guards the nest. When males become scarce, up to 5% of females raise their chicks with another female. After an extended courtship, they set up a nest.

Then they pull that same old lesbian trick. They sing to a male who already has a mate. Flaunting the promise of hot girl-on-girl action, they lure the male into their nest, use him for his sperm and then eject him. This frequently pisses off the adulterous male gull. Male ring-bills can be fierce fighters, and they are often stronger than females, but they are powerless against two lesbians defending a nest. Lesbians seem to have a thing about nests.

Lesbian female gulls in two-parent families raise chicks to adulthood in a way they never could if they were single moms. Biologists can see how, in at least two species of gulls, genes for lesbianism would enjoy selection advantage.

In any species where males kill each other in sufficient numbers, lesbianism can become a viable child-raising strategy. Glance at the nearest history textbook and see if you see any evidence of *Homo sapiens* males depleting their numbers fighting over territory, resources, and wombs. What's a girl to do? Or rather, who? Since most *Homo sapiens* sex serves more to bond than to procreate, girl-on-girl pair-bonding might have conferred a reproductive advantage to single-mom widows. Attend a campus party at Wellesley if you want to know what straight-A girls do when there are no males around. Worst place I've ever gone to pick up chicks.

If females made this secret known to the warriors, they could shut down human warfare. "Hey, Sergeant Fury, want to fight for this plot of land, or sneak home and watch the missus get it on with the maid?" To bring about world peace, we just need to understand male motivation.

Girl geese sometimes become third wheels to passionate love affairs between gay guy geese. Some of you ladies know the story: the gay geese like to hang out with her, but they invariably ignore her when they court each other with grand displays. But females find ways to get those gay genes. Once things get stud-hot, she literally dives between them to try and get herself fertilized, and in all the excitement she often succeeds. If she gets pregnant, next season you will see the three-parent family sharing food on the shores: a mother, a gaggle of goslings, and two dads.

Breeders of bovines who need sperm samples are always on the alert for hot lesbian action among cows. Why? Because it frequently causes erections in bulls. Bulls watch the cow cunnilingus for a while and then the farmer moves in to finish them off. Midwestern cow breeders treat female-on-female mounting as a respectable way to get bulls ready to produce calves, yet rarely use the method in their personal lives.

A large study of orcas included some passages about homosexual behavior among males. The US Marine Mammal Commission purchased the paper, deleted only the passages that mention homosexuality, and released it as a government report.

This is obviously the work of the Heterosexual Conspiracy. This cabal controls the government, the churches, and the schools, and they turn zoological reports into propaganda for their secret heterosexual agenda.

If you're laughing, they've gotten to you, too. This is no joke. Bruce Bagemihl, author of *Biological Exuberance: Animal Homosexuality and Natural Diversity* (St. Martin's Press, 1999) describes how persistently wildlife biologists on the front lines describe gay sex among animals as "greeting," "appeasement," and "dominance ritual."

A big group of male walruses meet, jump into a big pile, and engage in several minutes of enthusiastic rubbing, moaning, and licking. "Greeting behavior," says the biologist. I don't know why a friendly hello had to involve getting covered in ejaculate, but it can't be gay sex, since male lions do it, too. C'mon, there's no way the King of the Beasts is gay. It's "appeasement."

Ph.D. scholars have a proud history of phrasing their reports as incomprehensibly as possible. Writing about chimp testicles and walrus orgies and somehow making it boring is a skill that requires years of academic training. Tragically, I was never trained in scientific narcoleptic speak. I'm afraid I'll have to report it as a normal person. Bear with me.

Macho savanna baboon males say hello by stroking each other's scrotums. They also mount, nuzzle rumps, and kiss genitals. To the untrained eye, this might look like "affection." Biologists know it's dominance behavior. Though some gays I know refuse to accept the distinction.

In the United States' most revered and conservative animal institutions, homosexuality among rams runs rampant. A study of domesticated rams found that 16% refused to mate during mating season. Six percent seemed uninterested in sex at all. Ten percent were interested in sex only with other males. Ram, indeed.

Even sheep, those paragons of purity, have tendencies. To quote Rex Wockner, who wrote a piece reprinted in the book *Out in All Directions: The Almanac of Gay and Lesbian America, Vol. 1* (Warner Books, 1995): "Eight percent of the male sheep at the United States Department of Agriculture's Sheep Experimental Station in Dubois, Idaho, are gay." These sheep have anal intercourse—in public! The biggest social problem in the gay sheep community is that most gay male sheep want to be tops, and have trouble finding bottoms. Gay sheep bottoms are exceptionally popular at the Department of Agriculture.

With all the awe biologists have mustered to describe tool use, how come nobody mentions dildos? Primates invest time and effort into sculpting sex toys. Macaques have never been too bright when it comes to using tools to acquire termites or break open nuts. Yet one female macaque demonstrated five different sex toy designs she used solely for her own pleasure. Again, you have to understand female motivation: termites or orgasm?

Who needs a boyfriend when you've got a tail? Female Japanese macaques *love* their tails; though they have to clean them a lot more often. Primatologists are still exploring why they bother to fashion sex toys when they are born attached to their own personal vibrator.

Those who are born with less inviting tails have to innovate.

Female porcupines pork pine cones and straddle sticks. Then male porcupines masturbate on the same reeking sticks. I guess being covered in spikes really does make you kinkier.

Antlers are erogenous zones. Male deer rub their antlers against trees until climax. Dolphins rub their genitals against the sea bed, the tank floor, turtles, sharks, eels (not the electric kind), and the humans trying to study them. Male dolphins stick it in each other's blowholes. Female dolphins use their vaginas as suction cups to pick up objects. If our female ancestors had learned this trick, we might never have evolved hands.

Imagine if you couldn't talk. You're sitting around with your friends all day, naked. There's no TV, no magazines, no religion, no walls for privacy, nothing but food and bodies. What do you do to kill the time?

If my dog is any example, animals must be getting themselves and each other off at an amazing rate.

Now I feel ripped off by every nature show I ever saw. *Mutual of Omaha's Wild Kingdom* could have been a lot more wild and mutual. That's what happens when an insurance company in Omaha controls nature documentaries.

That's not the only TV show controlled by the insidious Heterosexual Conspiracy. Take a look at the *Discovery Channel*. These guys have no problem telling our children about straight male bears killing infant cubs and raping their mothers. Is lesbian love and parenting supposed to be a bigger threat to our children?

If the only natural sex is procreative sex, it sure is the rarest form of sex. Our species has mostly non-procreative sex. There is sex after menopause, sex during menstruation, sex during pregnancy, sex while lactating, oral sex, and sex with someone of the same sex. The all-time most frequent form of *Homo sapiens* sex?

The sex you just had. You know what I'm talking about: sex with your favorite lover.

And why is this? Why would evolution select for sexual behavior that doesn't produce offspring? Evolution knows darn well you can't impregnate yourself. That option is saved for snails and wheat. Where do you get off pleasing yourself?

It's time to understand a sophisticated concept in gene theory. To elucidate this subtle abstraction, we must closely analyze one key case study: your inability to stop masturbating.

Evolution doesn't design anything for a purpose. Evolution by chance designed erogenous zones, because erogenous zones by chance led to procreation. It doesn't mean any creature born with these pleasure mechanisms must use them for procreation. Natural selection created your genitals. Your genitals do not have to serve natural selection if you don't want them to.

My hands were not designed to type on a keyboard. Yet I'm using my hands for typing right now. And that's a good thing.

Evolution gave me hands because they *used to* lead to procreation. That doesn't mean evolution gave me hands *in order to* cause more procreation. Natural selection is a blind designer with no plan. It designs things with no point. We choose the point.

In Catholic school, I was taught that masturbation could blind a sinner. Science has since proven that regular sexual satisfaction is good for your health. Take a look at my picture on the back flap. I'm seventy-three.

Your genitals were built because they bonded your ancestors to other people, and secondarily because they made more people. Meanwhile, there they are, just sitting there, twenty-four hours a day.

What do you do to kill the time? Let's inspect a pair of boobies.

35.

Boobies

Ha! That title was chosen just to attract the attention of straight men and lesbians. Believe it or not, I'm going to tell you all you need to know about boobies without mentioning a single woman.

Blue-footed boobies, like bower birds, build nests out of sand for no other purpose than to impress mates. After sex, boobies generally tear down their love pads and build something more appropriate for children. Boobies do a lot of "lekking," which is biologese for strutting your stuff for the babes.

The courtship begins when one booby cruises past a nest. If the host seems interested, the cruiser lands and flashes his blue feet. If the host keeps watching, the cruiser points his beak toward the sky, spreads his wings, puffs out his chest, and whistles. The host's response is typically to bury the beak in the plumage. They climb into the nest, wherefrom can be heard groaning and whistling. The mating is done mostly from behind.

As part of my research, I went on a personal safari to study other lekking species. I didn't get any funding. For some reason being a fiction writer with no Ph.D. doesn't earn you any scientific standing. I had to finance my own safari. I loaded up my car with scientific instruments and drove five miles to Baker Beach in San Francisco.

Gay men, like bower birds and boobies, build nests out of sand for no other purpose than to attract mates. Baker Beach is honeycombed with the unique fortresses of this lekking animal. The courtship begins when a cruiser flashes some body part from his car. It's usually not his feet. If the host seems interested, the cruiser approaches the sand fort for a closer inspection. Just before they enter the nest, the cruiser generally points his penis toward the sky and thrusts out his chest. This time the host whistles, and often buries the beak in the plumage. They enter the sand nest, wherefrom can be heard groaning and giggling, though no more whistling.

I crept closer out of scientific curiosity. Immediately, I had to take evasive action as the specimens displayed their courtship rituals at me. At first I was embarrassed and annoyed. Didn't my safari hat give them any hints that I was here for research purposes? But so many gentlemen callers before had never so flamboyantly courted me, and soon I was trying out the female booby-wiggle. I fluffed my feathers and waddled my haunches. The courtship calls came to an abrupt end. Oh, well. Back to the data-collecting.

When the creatures are done with mating, they abandon their nests and gather in the parking lot with females of the species. I tried to join in on the witty banter, but the females seemed more interested in the gay men, who are always wit wizards, damn them. Something about my spying had made the gay men taciturn in my presence. I backed away slowly, observed quietly for an afternoon, and I have reached my conclusion.

To have the body of Rock Hudson, the wardrobe of Elton John, the hygiene of Liberace, the wit of Oscar Wilde, dozens of adoring women fans, and not use these gifts to coax women into bed seems to me criminally insane. To say nothing of having sex in sand.

When people insist that homosexuality is a choice, I'm hearing that they must have homosexual feelings. I certainly didn't experience my own heterosexuality as a choice. I didn't grow into boyhood, survey the various options, and say, "Yup, I think I'm gonna be straight." I was minding my own business, playing with my trucks, when all of a sudden Suzie Plimpton walked by and I said, "Woooooooow!" I knew I was supposed to hate her. I had hated her yesterday. Everything I knew told me she was positively cootie-infested. Yet, for no logical reason I could see, suddenly I really, really, really wanted to touch her. What was wrong with me? Did I *want* cooties?

For several years of grammar school, I experienced my arising heterosexuality as a shameful secret no one must ever know. No one had ever felt this way in the history of civilization, except sissies. The spontaneous gymnastics of my penis were obviously something I would have to see a doctor about. I fought it with everything I had, but finally I had to admit it to myself: I was a heterosexual. It took me several years of shame to muster the courage to come out.

There was no power on earth that could make me "choose" to find Billy the snot-shooter attractive. Granted, his skill with snot-shots was appealing. I envied his spit-in-the-air-and-catch-it-in-his-mouth trick. When I tried it, I always got spit shrapnel on my face. I couldn't quite achieve the loogie cohesion that Billy could. Billy was clearly a character worth emulating. I wanted to hang around with him. I liked him. I did not want to touch him, though. And suddenly, our quest to nauseate the girls at any cost seemed like a bad idea. It contradicted everything I believed in, but now it seemed like the girls were right. We were the ones who had cooties.

Now, I'm a grown-up. Men universally have cooties. If my buddy's knee touches me under the table, I get a reaction like when a girl in second grade touched me. "Eeeeew!" Whatever the opposite of cooties is, women have that. They have reverse cooties.

When that guy in the cowboy hat on *Jerry Springer* (which I watch as an anthropologist) tells me he beats up gays because they are making a criminal choice, I'm hearing that he has homosexual feelings that he is choosing to deny, and he's mad at people who make the other choice. I don't feel any need to beat up gay people— hey, it leaves more females for me—nor do I feel the compulsion to wear a cowboy hat indoors.

And I couldn't help noticing that, in the Baker Beach honey-combs, a cowboy hat works even better than a safari hat.

Shouldn't straight men thank gay men? The fact that all the best-looking, best-dressed guys turn out to be gay is a great thing. It means straight women have no choice but to date guys like me. I am in full support of as many men as possible converting to homosexuality, causing a great desperate flocking of straight women toward broke writers.

When my housemates read this chapter, they approved of the stereotype that gay men are better-looking, better-dressed, and wit-tier than I am, but they pretended to gag when I mentioned Liberace, Elton John, and Rock Hudson. This list, they said, is a typ-ical straight guy's idea of hip homosexual men. "Well, who is cooler than they are?" I demanded. They said if I want to understand why

they steal the attention of every woman I'm trying to date, I'd better do some research.

Out of self-interest, I conducted a scientific study of the people
who put the homo back in *Homo sapiens*.

36.

Homo *Homo sapiens*

Many transsexuals report experiencing the deep intuition that they have had the wrong bodies ever since they were six. The personal reports are powerful. Transsexuals often describe their bodies as a "mask" they are forced to wear.

D.F. Swaab, from the Graduate School of Neuroscience Amsterdam, dissected the brains of male-to-female transsexuals at the Netherlands Institute for Brain Research, and found that male transsexuals have a female structure in their brains.

Your reptilian hypothalamus is in charge of sexual behavior. Next time you get moist or erect, remember to thank your hypo-thalamus. Inside the hypothalamus is the *stria terminalis* [BSTc], which is known on the streets as the BST nucleus, and it's about the size of a grain of rice. Males typically have BST nuclei that are

50% bigger than those of females. Women are short-grain. Men are long-grain. That's what makes us men. It doesn't matter if you're straight or gay. If you're male, your BST rice grain is on average 50% bigger than a female's.

Except for male transsexuals.

By some estimates, one person in 350,000 believes he or she was born with the wrong gender. After dissecting eleven brains of transsexuals—males who claimed they "felt female" ever since childhood—and comparing them with other brains, Swaab found that transsexuals—and *only* transsexuals—have BST nuclei that are the same size as females. As researchers said in their study: "The size of the BSTc was not influenced by sex hormones in adulthood, and was independent of sexual orientation."

Swaab said, "Our results indicate that other structures in the brain could be involved," and that this was the "tip of the iceberg." Swaab suspects there is "a whole network of cells and fibers connecting them, and we've only found the first one."

The little rice-grain in our big brains might be analogous to the little island of England that ruled the whole globe. If your body looks male, yet you feel like a woman, don't fret. A tiny empire in your brain that rules your sexuality looks just like a woman's. As far as your hypothalamus is concerned, you are a woman, penis or no penis.

So, male-to-female transsexuals have a uniquely female brain structure. Do gay men have brain structures unique to them?

Dr. Simon LeVay, a neurobiologist at the Salk Institute in La Jolla, California, became a reluctant celebrity overnight when he compared and contrasted another structure in the hypothalamus that "regulates male-typical sex behavior." It's one millimeter big. Brain scientists gave this locus of male virility the sexy name INAH3.

It turns out the INAH3 in heterosexual men is, *on average*, two to three times as big as a female's. The INAH3 in homosexual men is, *on average*, the same size as a female's.

LeVay, a gay man himself, said, "I am saying that gay men have a women's INAH3—they've got a woman's brain in that particular part."

LeVay became the center of a political storm. Any hate or fan mail you can imagine came to his mailbox. Homophobes loved him. Gays loved him. Homophobes hated him. Gays hated him. People thanked him for exonerating homosexuals. People derided him for being a self-hating homosexual. People said he vanquished the religious right. People said he armed the religious right.

Note that I italicized "on average" above. Therein lies the *scientific* criticism of this finding. LeVay found a range of INAH3 sizes in male brains. Most of the biggest INAH3s were on straight men. Most of the smallest INAH3s were on gay men. But there was broad overlap over a continuum of sizes. If you see an INAH3 in the middle range, there's no way to tell if that brain is straight or gay.

But this criticism gels with the notion that there are gradations of sexual orientation. Is sexuality a continuum analogous to the range in INAH3 sizes?

And why is all the most suggestive research coming from the study of male brains? I'm sure women have no problem with a systematic study of male brains, but where is all the lesbian data? Are women getting the shaft once again?

The answer to these questions lies in ancient females, who've been around four times longer than males. Males have only been around a little more than a billion years. Ancient females developed maleness along a slow continuum.

If you took honors biology class, you might remember being

forced to learn Ernst Haeckel's biological dictum: "Ontogeny recapitulates phylogeny."

This is fancy-pants geek speak that means: fetal development replays evolution. Before unborn babies look like humans, they look like monkeys. Before that, they look like amphibians. Before that, they have gills and fins. Before that, they look like worms. Way back at the beginning of fetal development, every organism looks like a female.

This does not mean males are an evolutionary upgrade from females. It means females invented males to better facilitate their own reproduction. Females are the first sex, and males are the second sex. God did not fashion woman from man's rib. A primeval sisterhood fashioned males from females' ribosomes.

Ribosomes are the numerous molecular engines in every cell that build organisms one molecule at a time, using only twenty amino acids as materials, and reading gene instructions coded into DNA. Hear that? They just welded another protein into your fingernail. Ribosomes are the hard-hats who keep a steady construction project going on in your body. For about three billion years, the whole business was run by females.

Way back in the days when everybody was a single-cell female, we cloned daughters by splitting in half. When it became a reproductive advantage to trade genes between individuals, we started sex, which caused more diversity. Some offspring were smaller, others bigger. This made sexual competition interesting. Females gave orders to the ribosome factories to create some smaller offspring that sacrificed nutrients for mobility. These were males. Suddenly single-cell females didn't want to be single any more. They wanted to make offspring using male genes. Females invented males to transport genes among each other.

Notice how, right from the beginning, males are more mobile, aggressive, and hungry, and females are more stationary, receptive, and equipped with nutrients. It's to the male's advantage to be indiscriminate, and it's in the female's interests to be choosy.

It also means all males must be built from female body plans. There are many steps along this process of development, and not all males take all the steps toward maleness, and some females take a step or two in the male direction.

37.

Why Males and Females Don't Actually Exist

There's actually no such thing as a gender. There are really six billion human genders, each aligned across a continuum, with a statistical bunching at either the male end or the female end. If you were to graph it out, with one side male and the other side female, you would see a big U. Most people fall somewhere on the extreme ends. A significant minority of people range somewhere in between, like Jerry Springer's cowboy guy. Since no restaurant wants to build six billion bathrooms, they just say "Men's" and "Women's" and let us work it out.

Are you having trouble deciding whether you are a man or a woman? Your genitals are only part of the story. To be a male or a female, you can't just waltz up and say, "I have a penis! Let me into the tree house!" or "Here's my vagina! Let's go shopping!"

Slow down. To be a male or a female, you need a whole range of body parts and mental gadgets. Many men don't have all the male parts, and many females don't have all the female parts, and lots of us have a few of each, all interacting in our brains.

For instance, I have female parts in my brain.

Look at me. I look like a typical guy. I act like a typical guy. I'm good at guy stuff. I can catch and throw. I'm good with directions. I came out of the womb knowing how to barbecue. How can plaid not "match" with plaid when they're the same damn thing? What the hell is "ambiance" anyway? She's got a lot of nerve saying I'm rude for watching the game while she's talking. She's the one talking while I'm trying to watch the game.

But during all this research into evolutionary biology, I took some of the tests that show male-female cognitive differences, and I discovered something disturbing:

I have a female brain.

I have a penis! I swear! So let's just establish this firmly and masculinely: I definitely have a penis. Trust me, I checked several times while I took the tests.

It all started when I got bored with reading academic literature and busted into *The Brain Pack: An Interactive, Three-Dimensional Exploration of the Mysteries of the Mind*, by Ron Van der Meer and Ad Dudink (Running Press, 1996). I knew this had to be informative, because Van der Meer was the same guy who did the *Sesame Street* pop-up books. (Hey, it's *fun*, okay?)

First, I took the test that women are supposed to be good at. Let's see, which of these color patterns fades into another one exactly like the example? Well, obviously, that one has the subtle shading from periwinkle to aquamarine to turquoise to cornflower blue, and those don't. I must be getting this one wrong, because it's too easy. Now I'm supposed to figure out this equation in my head. Again, it seems too easy. Are you trying to tell me most guys can't get this? Which of these items match with those items? Obvious! Which of these pictures has one tiny detail different from the others? Simple!

It took me half a minute. I checked the answer key. Perfect score. This obviously proves that men are superior. I can't wait to show this to my girlfriend. Scientific proof that I'm always right!

Then I took the test that men are supposed to excel in. This should be a snap. Wait. All these are the same three-dimensional shapes only turned around? They look like different shapes to me. I'll guess B. If I poke this folded paper with holes, then unfold it; I'm supposed to predict where all the holes will be on the unfolded paper. What am I, an expert in origami now? Why is the test for men so much harder? Uh-oh, an abstract word problem! I hate these! How many bushels am I supposed to sell over the next twelve days to make up a 20% loss of—what? I'll guess C.

It took me five minutes. I checked the answer key. I got a third of them wrong. Another third I got purely on lucky guesses.

I can't do male mental tasks!

Even worse, I excel at female mental tasks. I definitely have to cut down on the Luna bars.

Let's try the maze. Ha! I navigated the whole thing in under a minute! Beat that, girls! My mental masculinity is restored!

Then I checked the answer key. Women do the maze by memorizing landmarks. Men typically do the maze by geometrical reasoning and don't even notice the landmarks. I can't remember the abstract shape of my route, but I remember every item in the maze.

I closed the test book with red ears. My brain has no balls.

I sprinted home from the library, changed into flannel and work boots, lifted some weights, ordered red meat and beer. I was disassembling my car engine when it hit me: I can perform feats most of my fellow men can't.

"Cool!" I thought. "I have a female brain! That's why I have so many women friends and can stay up all night talking! That's why I'm intuitive and sensitive and such a good listener! Maybe I can use this to get sex!" (I didn't say *all* my brain parts were female.)

Back on the Pleistocene savanna, I'd be the guy who got lost while hunting, screeched when I heard the charging boar, and accidentally threw my spear at Grok. My fellow hunters beat me up, made me cry, and sent me home, where I excelled at baby-sitting, sewing stylish patterns, and sensitive listening. Then when the jocks went off to chase down another giant carnivorous bear, I diddled their wives, swelled the size of their testicles, and passed on my girly-boy genes.

What's fascinating to me isn't my scores. What's fascinating is that I experienced all the female questions as easy, obvious. All the male questions were difficult. They made me furrow my brow. They gave me a headache.

Reading up on all these male and female cognitive tests, I found the most entertaining part was reading about one gender's reaction to the other gender's performance. It's not just that men and women find their tests easy, it's that they can't see how the other sex can't see it!

Among the Ache, feminine men are called *panegi*. Loosely translated, it means wuss. *Panegi* don't hunt, but weave and gather with the girls. Other Ache men taunt them and make them the butt of dirty jokes. If Ache men get extra surviving offspring by being hunters of great prowess, how do genes for *panegi* keep cropping up?

It is a mystery the brave hunters must wonder about as they head off on their business trips, and leave the women and *panegi* at home.

I spent five years being the only male nanny in the Bay Area: a "manny." Moms and kids loved me. Dads tolerated me. For every one hundred parents who wanted a female babysitter, there was one little boy who was sick and tired of all these female caretakers and wanted somebody who would wrestle with him. I cornered that market, moms started recommending me to other moms, and my baby-sitting career ran itself, especially once I offered my free consultation on why, when it comes to hallways with too much sunlight, peach just doesn't work like primrose to add a sense of flow.

It looks like most of my observable body parts are male, and most of my observable behavior is male, but some of my cognitive talents are better suited to gathering nuts and baby-sitting kids.

About 90% of women have brains wired for female behavior. About 10% of women have masculinized brains. About 10% from this group are lesbians.

It's estimated that 80% to 85% of men have brains wired for male behavior, and 15% to 20% of men have feminized brains. Some of these men are gay.

These are very rough estimates, culled from a variety of sources, but it looks like men might be twice as likely to be femme as women are to be butch.

What percentage of Americans in general is gay? Again we must rely on polls like the ones we use to determine the president's approval rates, which are rough estimates at best. From these we can estimate that 4% to 5% of men and 2% to 4% of women are predominantly homosexual most of their lives. The 2000 U.S. census determined how many gay couples live together as committed partners, and by extrapolation the proportion of homosexuals in the population was figured to be 2.5% of men and 1.2% of women.

The two-to-one disparity remains consistent across many esti-mates even though about 7.5% of both sexes admit to experiencing sexual attraction to the same sex. Gary J. Gates co-authored *The Gay & Lesbian Atlas*, and he says women's conception of their own sexu-ality is more fluid than men's, so women are less liable to label their desires with an identity. Interestingly, about three-quarters of trans-sexuals are men who want to be women (about 60,000 in the U.S.A.) and about one-quarter are women who want to be men.

Researchers at UCLA have identified fifty-four genes involved in determining a person's sexuality. Those genes can be turned on and off in many combinations to create your unique sexual disposition.

How could we all range along a gender rainbow like this? Aren't we supposed to be breeding? Why doesn't nature make half of us male and half of us female and be done with it?

Well, first of all, we all start out as female.

38.

Why Men Have Nipples

Judging by the mind-numbing studies of chimp testicles, many scientists seem to believe there is in inverse proportion between humor and rigor. My scientist buddies frown at my chapter called "Why Men Have Nipples" and say it should be entitled something like, "Adaptive Significance of Male Nipplosity as Phylogenic Baggage."

But the grandfather of biology, as far as I am concerned, is Aristotle, who asserted that everything in biology has a point. His student Theophrastus, in the scientific spirit of spite, cited men's nipples as an example of uselessness.

These are the minds that I keep company with, not my biologist colleagues with their so-called "degrees." Aristotle didn't have a Ph.D. Neither do I. Coincidence? Aristotle used straightforward language, whereas most of what scientists say is all Greek to me.

The master template of all organisms is female. Human embryos, for the first month of gestation, develop more or less as females. Then around week seven, right when we are a centimeter long, embryos that inherit a Y-chromosome are pickled in a series of hormonal brews, each changing something new in the embryo to a male. The primevally female embryo is slowly masculinized by a timed series of hormone waves.

One wave changes something in the genitals and the brain; another changes something else in the brain; then a third; then more. Most of these baths happen before birth, and mostly affect the brain. Another hormonal tsunami hits at puberty, which primarily changes the body. Any *in utero* hormone surge that does not take, does not change that one aspect of the embryo to a male orientation.

Listen up, tomboys. Sometimes girls in the womb are exposed to male hormones. Numerous studies, like those of Anke Ehrhardt of Columbia University, show that girls with excess exposure to male androgens in the womb exhibit more aggression than their sisters. Studies by S.A. Berenbaum and others found that when given a choice of toys, these girls consistently chose balls over books, demolition over dolls, building houses over playing house. They played with toy cars as long as boys did. These girls performed better than other girls at spatial tests, object-rotation tests, and finding shapes in a pattern—all tests that boys usually excel in. They were also good at grand hand-eye coordination—like a boy playing catch—and bad with minute hand-eye coordination—like a girl executing perfect handwriting or threading a needle.

Some of them can also kick your ass. Girls exposed to testosterone in the womb expend higher levels of energy during play, choose boys as playmates, initiate more fights, have fewer fantasies of motherhood, almost no interest in dolls, are grossed out by infant care, and prefer functional clothes to attractive clothes.

What's fascinating is that these little girls even choose against many feminine qualities that they clearly get from their culture, like jewelry, make-up, and hairstyling. In many cultures, macho men wear make-up and jewelry, style their hair, and dress more colorfully, while women wear functional clothes. If men and women's choices vary across cultures, they're probably not biological. If men and women's choices are universal across cultures, they probably are biological.

These girls were told they were girls, had the genitalia of girls, yet instinctively felt that they should reject accoutrements typically associated with girls. All because of one little testosterone bath in the womb.

Tragic genetic mistake? Nope. The continuum of human sexuality is so consistent that we should think of people who end up somewhere in the middle—the No Man's Land of transgender—as viable gene reproduction strategies that Mother Nature has found successful. We could say butch girls and femme boys are part of nature's plan—if nature had a plan. It's more accurate to say that in the competition to survive and reproduce, butch girls and femme boys are winners. Otherwise they wouldn't be here in such large numbers.

The timed series of hormone waves isn't rigidly set, like clockwork. It improvises new game plans. Some primevally female embryos change entirely into males. Others are genetically coded to stop somewhere in the middle. In other cases, environmental factors that affect the mother can change the delicate titration of hormones in her womb.

An embryo that received some waves of testosterone, but skipped one, might become male in most ways, but not all ways.

Maybe he didn't get the testosterone surge that would have made him attracted to women, given him the ability to turn shapes in his head, and suppressed any chance for a flair for interior decoration. And something about Katharine Hepburn is just so cool.

An embryo with no Y chromosome that didn't get any testosterone baths except one, might be female in most ways, but not all ways. Maybe that one testosterone bath gave her an attraction to other girls and a compulsion to tell jokes in public places—and there is something about rugby she finds irresistible.

The straight woman, frustrated with her boyfriend's inability to understand how she feels, who goes to her gay male friend for consolation, might not be reacting to the ways culture trains gay and straight men to be different. One male might have received an *in utero* hormone surge that made him less emotionally intuitive, but better at geometrical reasoning. The other male might not have received that particular *in utero* hormonal surge, so in the areas of emotional intuition and machinery fascination, he is female. Females recognize female qualities in each other, just like straight men are comfortable hanging around with other straight men, and gay men are comfortable hanging around with gay men, and lesbians hang out in big groups. We have an intuitive recognition of sameness. However we officially deny it, it's how most of us operate in the world.

During our stay in the womb, there are several different hormone tides to choose from. Some of us have genes that treat these *in utero* options as a buffet: "I'll take the penis, the engineering talent, and the beard, but I'd rather not have the one that makes me aggressive, please." *Voila!* Sensitive New Age guy is born.

Another fetus says: "I don't want the Y chromosome, so I get the vagina, the waist-to-hip ratio, a creepy telepathy that tells me precisely what my boyfriend is hiding, and zero ability to find my own damn way to the airport, but I'll take whatever hyena-style testosterone surge that gives me aggression, the inability to admit I'm wrong, and the female hyena's need to make males grovel in the dirt for sex." *Voila!* My girlfriend is born.

These hormonal tides are timed to influence our choices. Most occur inside the womb, but other hormone changes happen during the course of our lives. Puberty prepares us for the dating games. Men's testosterone levels start to dip after thirty-five when a shift from mating to parenting is necessary. Women become extra horny at thirty-five as fertility starts to lessen. Men have mid-life crises at fifty when their fertility starts to lessen. Women go through sudden menopause at fifty when pregnancy becomes too dangerous and a grandmother's lore is necessary to tribe survival. All these crises are controlled by timed hormone changes in the body that were set up on the Pleistocene savanna. They are sacraments we all must receive. Some of us just do it more gracefully than others.

In a species where most members are all male or all female, it looks like a minority of strategies ended up somewhere in between and contributed to the survival of the human family. In nature, diversity is an asset.

Now you know why men have nipples. Men are fundamentally female—just souped-up with fancy accoutrements.

Now I'm going to give you some scientific data that will make all the women love me, and all the men hate me. But to hell with men! Who needs them, right, ladies? All you women need is one guy who is willing to sell out his fellow guys to support women's liberation! That's where I come in! (Every man supports feminism to the extent he thinks it will get him laid.)

There are scattered bits of evidence that suggest your husband can breast-feed.

You just leaned closer to this page, didn't you?

If men drink enough alcohol, they lactate. The liver suppresses our female hormones, yet females produce enough to get past the liver. But if men damage their liver with too many manly quaffs of Budweiser, our embarrassing little secret becomes apparent. Your guy will start lactating like a male Dayak fruit bat. Inside every man is a woman trying to get out.

Another way to make a man lactate is to starve him, then feed him. At the end of World War II, 500 prisoners of war were liberated from Japanese concentration camps. When suddenly well-fed after years of starvation, they grew breasts and lactated. Their female hormones kicked in before their livers recovered from malnutrition and shut that nonsense down.

I know I'm supposed to report only the scientific data, but I am also from a gossipy species. There are unconfirmed claims floating around out there—of the South American tribe where men attach infants to their nipples and lactate within six weeks; of sensitive American men who attach themselves to a breast pump for a few months until they start to lactate; of men who empathize so deeply with their woman's pregnancy they not only experience labor contractions, but lactate on cue. Look into this, ladies. If women can become athletes, CEOs, and lumberjacks, men can take a turn breast-feeding. Why not? You're the sex that invented males. Remember, men are only men titularly.

If men are women in hormonal disguise, shouldn't egg-makers and sperm-makers be getting along swimmingly? Of course. The problems sperm and eggs cause us are only a secondary side effect of the deeper, ancient sperm and egg solution.

39.

The Sperm and Egg Solution

Most organisms reproduce by splitting in half. Some organisms evolved sex. Sex is gene-combining.

In the single-cell realm, males are little, mobile, and hungry. Females are large, less mobile, and have nutrients. This means males must impregnate, and females must get pregnant.

Add a half-billion years of evolution, and you get multi cellularity. Males make plentiful sperm. Females make rare eggs. Sperm must compete for eggs, and eggs make sperm compete for them. This means males are indiscriminate, and females are choosy.

Males have a higher chance of reproducing a whole lot or never reproducing at all. This makes males more competitive and aggressive and power-mad. Females have a good chance of reproducing, but since they reproduce fewer offspring, they have less chance of their few offspring surviving. This makes females more safety-conscious and parental, yet more attracted to the victorious and powerful.

Then, our species came up with a unique problem, which is something our species excels at. Our brains are big and must be built outside the womb, which means children take forever to grow up, which means big-brained parents have to pair-bond for a very long time to make a nest. The nuclear family is a kind of secondary womb.

Men and women are different in so many subtle ways, but all their innate differences come from very simple evolutionary principles.

Men don't get pregnant. Women do.

This means men are more mobile, and women tend to be stationary.

This means men become hunters, and women become gatherers.

This means men's brains focus, and women's brains multitask.

This means arguments in the nest.

Sperm-makers want to spread sperm around. Egg-makers want the very best sperm. This means arguments during the date.

Humans who can't get pregnant want the best receptacle for their sperm. Humans who do get pregnant want the best helper with their nest. This means after we finish arguing, we have sex.

Sex means babies. Babies mean more arguing.

Our species specializes in compromise. Without compromise between men and women specializing in different tasks, our species would have gone extinct. This means men and women, despite having different reproductive interests, evolve to crave compromise to make a nest. We are genetically programmed to fall in love.

When most humans in most cultures choose to hang out with

somebody, they generally hang out with people of their own sex. The *same* sex is always the *sane* sex. Why would anybody want to spend their lives with a member of that weird other sex? Especially when time spent with them leads to time spent with the most childish people of all: children. Biology finds a way to trick you into making this insane choice. It's called love.

Who is in charge? You or your genes?

If you're still laboring under the delusion that you're in control, not your genes, wait until you fall in love or become a parent. Let's define love biologically: Love is when your genes kick your ass.

We have selfish genes, which makes us tend toward selfishness. I could have given a buck to that hungry, homeless schizophrenic today, but instead I spent it on extra syrup in my mocha latte. I wouldn't go out of my way to hurt that poor guy, but I wouldn't go out of my way to help him, either. I go out of my way to avoid him.

I don't love him. I love my mocha latte. My tongue rewards me with pleasure when it detects the extra calories that will help me store even more fat for the famine that will never come. That's more important to me than helping some non-kin non-friend non-cute person in a real famine.

Then, after coffee I'll attend church, so I can save my own ass in the afterlife. Church is like a weekly investment in an IRA for retirement. I'd rather invest one hour a week in my own salvation in the next world, than one hour a week nurturing orphans in this world.

You think you're better than me? Your brain isn't. My typing "mocha latte with extra syrup" just put you in the mood for a mocha latte with extra syrup. It did not put you in the mood to spend that money on a homeless, hungry schizophrenic who isn't cute. You might buy a mocha latte tomorrow. You probably won't accompany an orphan to church tomorrow.

When genes need to get the hell out of me, they change my program. Love is what happens when I care about somebody else more than myself. Love is our most important passion, because love is when selfish genes move on from us, into the future we will never see. Our love of self exists in service to selfless love.

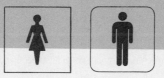

40.

Falling in Love

I was born about the time rock stars stopped holding their guitars over their hearts and started holding them over their crotches. A great cultural shift occurred around the day of my birth. It changed our ideologies, social structures, and, tragically, our hair styles. It did not change our Pleistocene emotions. Historical cataclysms never do.

My roaring twenties ended with the Great Depression of my thirties. I had a crash at twenty-nine. My genes invested in the wrong woman.

Note that I say my genes, not "me." The rational me fought the feeling with everything I had. I stayed up all night arguing with it. But it didn't matter what my rational mind said. My irrational desire grabbed my rational mind by the lapels and growled, "From now on, you work for me! Get it?"

True love is not chosen. True love chooses you. Falling in love is something that happens to us. We can't help it.

Love is an overwhelming passion, because once you fall in love, your genes stop preserving you until you've spotted the optimum mate, and they start telling you, "Mate, pair-bond, right now, at all costs. This is what we built you for. Screw your friends, destroy your life, throw away your future, because now is our chance to get the hell out of your doomed body and into the next generation."

Our cells had past lives. Our ancestors possess us in our passions. We play out ancient dramas. We haven't forgotten our lines: I can't live without you. You complete me. Life is meaningless without you. I'll kill myself, your lover, or you if I can't have you. I mean it. I'm crazy with love. I'm out of control.

Clichés become clichés by virtue of their being true. What's eternally true about being human is the incantation of our genes. And they plan to stay eternal—even though they have no plan.

Gene designs ride our bodies like we're ships destined to sink. Their only way out is through our genitals. They'll trick us if they have to. Genes fill our brains with illusions:

"I know it seems like she's a college freshman, but really she is a genius of maturity. Sure, I'll lose my tenure, but which is more important, my career or love?"

"Just because he's married to her law firm doesn't mean he won't leave her and take me away from this cash register forever. Funny how I never noticed my own spouse is an agent of Satan before."

"Love this holy cannot be desecrated by a condom. All my friends who confronted me about this affair are hereby my enemies. They're just jealous. No one will ever understand how unique we are. In this history of the cosmos, nobody has ever loved the way we love."

You will occasionally hear postmodern historians say that chivalric troubadours in eleventh-century Provence invented the experience of romantic love. This is absolute crap. Pleistocene people fell madly in love long before medieval minstrels started prancing around in tights. Erotic love is a human universal, existing in some form in all 168 cultures studied. The anguish of love dominates most art, music, and poetry, everywhere. Falling in love is a sacrament coded into our genes. We can't get around it.

All living things blossom when it's time for courtship. Caterpillars turn to butterflies. Buds turn into flowers and fruit. You turn into an idiot. Females everywhere perfume the atmosphere and sprout fecundity announcements. Males turn into warriors with weapons growing from their heads and brightly colored flags sticking up from their tails or manes or genitals. All living things become ready to breed or die trying. It seems like it's what they were created for, their purpose in life.

But, there is no purpose in life. All biological beauty happens not *in order to* copy genes, but *because it happened* to copy genes in the past.

The gene reproduction strategy that happened to work for our species is love. That's why we act like love is something special. Once you go insane for another *Homo sapiens*, you transmogrify into the state your sanity was built for.

Petunias are very good at hiding, conserving energy, and surviving until it's time to trade genes, when all of a sudden they go crazy and become beautiful. All living things are conservative, efficient, safe, and drab until it's time to breed, at which point they become extravagant, wasteful, risky, and beautiful. The primary purpose of the sober state of being is to prepare for the impassioned state of being.

We *Homo sapiens* are very good at thinking clearly and surviving in a social context, until it's time to trade genes, at which point we go mad. The stupidity of our overwhelming passions comes from a deeper wisdom than anything the wise can control. The definition of passion: when you become animated by an ancient imperative that transcends your mortal life. Passion comes from before you were born, and it reaches out beyond your death. To a gene, your passions are more important than you. We celebrate that ecstatic agony in our art and gossip, because there is no state achievable by humans that is more self-transcendent.

Fools don't fall in love. Lovers only look like fools to the wise, because those who aren't in love are merely preserving their bodies and social structures until they or their relatives fall in love, so they have nothing better to do than be wise. He who is wise is reason's slave. "Reason is emotion for the sexless," said the actor and poet Heathcote Williams. "People who are sensible about love are incapable of it," said Douglas Yates. Bob Dylan said, "You can't be in love and wise at the same time."

I've stopped expecting love to make sense. "Sense" is the servant of its master. We are not the authors of our decisions. We are the rationalizers of our impulses. Our passions read from a script written in our DNA text. As John Lennon proved with his love of Yoko, love is not only blind but deaf.

Love, or erotic passion, sometimes overrides our passion for self-preservation. That's why *Romeo and Juliet* makes us sigh and cry. We know they're stupid teenagers. We know it won't last. We also remember we never felt so alive as when we were stupid teenagers in stupid love.

That's because teenagers hold the keys to the driving force behind human evolution. Many Pleistocene newborns struggled to focus on the faces of their teenage parents. Most humans got born because of the passionate impulses of young people, not the sober decisions of the mature. When it came to surviving on the savanna, teenage passion worked like a high-octane engine.

If we didn't have our neocortical ability to foresee scenarios and weigh consequences, there would be a lot more tragic stories. In harsher, poorer societies, people risk death for sexual passion much more readily. They look to their futures and don't see much worth preserving. Now is their only chance to live—which is really each gene screaming in divine chorus, "Get me the heck out of this mortal body! This is our last chance!"

Most art and gossip is not about the old and wise and responsible. Most art and gossip is about the young and foolish and impassioned. When characters struggling in stories attain the safe, enlightened, or married state of being, stories end, because drama stops. Stories end where conflicts are resolved. The only social event worth talking about is conflict.

Young people act young, and old people act old, because the way they act is the best strategy for the genes for which they encode. Older people want to preserve family stability and impart wisdom. Younger people want to assert their individuality and compete for attention to distinguish themselves from competing breeders.

Everybody's got a different job to do, and we all work for the same boss. The passionate die in much larger numbers than the sober. The passionate breed and bond faster than the sober. The sober maintain bonds they forged when they were passionate, so they can rear and guide little demons of passion.

Youth isn't wasted on the young. Passion is finished with the old.

Most animals die after they are finished being young and fertile. Our species produced elders because our tribes survive on information, and the brains of elders were once our internet, our encyclopedias. Sages are the servants of the breeders and the babies. And they know it. Elders are teachers by instinct. All elders are annoyed that the young don't listen. Elders enforce rules to guide the instincts of the young.

Youngsters live mainly in their emotional limbic systems, because hormones put them there. Elders live mainly in their rational neocortexes, because hormones put them there. Conflicts between the young and the old are the conflict between the hypo-thalamus and the neocortex, passion and reason.

There is only one type of person who is a bigger fool than a person in love: a parent. These people have lost all grasp on reality. As a daycare worker, I always had to bite my tongue before it said:

"Believe it or not, Mrs. Lubenow, Maurice didn't shove a gum-ball up his nose because he's sending you a subliminal message that he wants yet more of your attention. He shoved a gumball up his nose because Maurice is a moron. Let's face it, Mrs. Lubenow, all six-year-olds are."

If you want to see an educated adult act irrationally, vaguely imply that his kid is not the purpose of the universe—or, even bet-ter, imply that his kid *is* the purpose of the universe. (Hey, I knew how to get tips.)

Your brain is never really free of its long-term goal of copying your genes. Try to have an intimate conversation without referring to sexual passion. Try to tell a joke without referring to sexual desire. Lie down at night, close your eyes, and see if you think about anything but sexual passion. If you're a parent, close your eyes, look in your heart, and ask what you want most in the world. You'd sacrifice yourself to see your babies grown and healthy.

That's because your genes know that your babies, once they reach breeding age, are more important than you.

Decide to stop being in love. Choose to not love your kids. Tell yourself you will never be turned on again. Tell yourself to stop grieving a lost family member. Decide you don't need to sleep any more. Then ask yourself who is in charge, you or your genes.

When somebody you love is cruel to you, you may be able to transform love into hate, but you can't just turn passion off, flick the switch into indifference. I can't choose to make pain go away any more than I can choose to make love go away. Pain and love never listen to me. They give the orders, and I follow.

Your neocortex is the newcomer in your skull, and it's been arguing with your "heart" (meaning hypothalmus) ever since it showed up. Your neocortex was invented to steer your heart through a complicated community. Your heart has an ancient friendship with your genes. Your neocortex is an energy-expensive consultant, taken on board only recently, and it was designed to serve the imperatives of the gene, and the gene is as old as life itself. That's the only reason we can have high-flung thoughts at all.

Religious ceremony uses the language of courtship, and courtship uses the language of religious ecstasy. At orgasm, we cry out to God. Love makes us idealize lovers, rejection makes us demonize lovers, and we often never get to know the person in between. We think our love is written in the stars, because it is written in our genetic code.

Maybe I'm just an uncultured clod, but I look at Michelangelo's ceiling, and I see a gay man's erotic fantasies. The whole thing looks like a big ejaculation onto a ceiling. All Michelangelo's women look like men, all his breasts look wrong, and he loves to put faces near penises. Gay male artists depict naked men, and straight male artists depict naked women.

Renaissance paintings of Hell are orgies. Hieronymous Bosch is sadomasochistic porn, as are Swanenburgh and van Eyck. When these guys drew Hell, they drew their deepest desires: beautiful, young, naked bodies squirming around in piles and getting sodomized by devils. What a punishment! The damned are so passionate, they're on fire.

Signorelli's "The Damned Cast into Hell" makes me hot: devils chewing on ears and embracing the torsos of playmates who look a lot more passionate than pained. Everybody in Hell is extremely good-looking. Bernini's sculpture "The Ecstasy of St. Theresa" lives up to her sweaty account of what it's like to be pierced by an angel. Whoa, Nelly. Take a look at Pollaiuolo's sculpture "Hercules and Antaeus"—two gods wrestling with gratuitous crotch connection—and his "Battle of Ten Naked Men," which looks like a club in San Francisco due for a police raid.

And why a police raid? Why does every society punish sex?

Freud says religion and art flourish to the extent we repress sexual passion. But really, civilization flourishes to the extent we repress sexual passion. To found a civilization, sex must be controlled.

This is when men utilize the principle upon which every civilization is founded: The way women make us feel is their fault. They rob us of our *gravitas*. How are we supposed to run the world with all these exposed ankles bewitching us? Sexuality is a force for chaos, and the first thing any tribe does to organize itself is say, "We must control sex." The most significant differences among cultures on this planet are, at core, beliefs about how sex should be controlled.

Of course we're uptight. We *Homo sapiens* had better be. Humans need repression. People are afraid of sex, because sex is dangerous. Sex doesn't just make people. Sex kills people.

In modern hunter-gatherer societies, and in American inner cities, men murder men chiefly over women, at about the same per capita rate. Women scar, starve, and cripple themselves primarily in service to standards of beauty. Bound feet, anorexia, punctured flesh, ritualized scarring in Africa, self-cutting in the U.S.A., surgery to remove, surgery to add. When we are sexually scorned, men strike at other bodies, and women strike at their own bodies. Everybody is fighting to control the body that has the womb.

In every culture, the primary cause of murder is not money or drugs, but sex. That's right, sex is more dangerous than heroin. All heroin does is hijack the endrocronological system that rewards you for doing something that was reproductively advantageous for our ancestors. You are far more likely to be killed by a jealous lover than a stranger. You are far more likely to get addicted to love than heroin. And the withdrawal is brutal.

Sexuality is the primary reason some teenagers are included, other excluded. Rejecting sexual passion causes suicide. Who flirts with whom, hierarchies of attention that result, violent jealousy, consuming lust, and competition between rivals is scary and it gets out of control. Civilization is a structure that organizes these forces. It keeps us from killing each other like most *Homo sapiens* do when they don't have a civilization. Sex is powerful; sex is dangerous; sex matters more than anything in the world, except the results of sex. Sex invented love to make sure we rear our big-brained babies.

Without desire, there would be no man-made catastrophes. Erotic love tells you risks are worth it; hurting other people is worth it; destructive decisions are worth it. Invariably, we come out the other side a little older and with a more cynical viewpoint on romantic passion. We're proud of ourselves for gaining our wisdom about love, for knowing better, for using our elder power to control the foolish young. . .

. . .until Wave Two, when the mid-life crisis kicks in. Now we become the fools again, and our new beloved is all that matters. We'll destroy our whole life for her or him.

Everyone outside love looks inside and says it's a psychosis. It's not. It's as natural as the soberness of being a responsible adult. Anyone in love looks at his neighbors and sees zombies going through the motions. Anyone in love looks at his pre-love state and sees someone who wasn't really alive. Anyone with a broken heart looks at everybody else and sees people who enjoy their lives, while we will never know happiness again, and nobody will ever understand.

None of it counts as crazy. There is no sanity. The sane are people who agree with us. The "sane" are on our side, the "insane" are those we declare a right to control. Sanity is merely the pathology that functions. Change functions, change sanities. When you fall in love or make a baby, your function changes, and so do the physical structures of your body and brain.

Your mind physically changes according to the dictates of your glands. We are marionettes, and the puppet master is inside our bodies, using liquid strings of blood attached to our muscles and filigreed through each tiny gadget in our brains. Since our neocortexes were built by sociality and cooperation, humans need to connect with other hearts and minds. Nobody needs to connect like family—except men or women in love. Family shares your genes. Lovers might pass on your future genes. Friends form alliances of affection to aid each other in communities where we compete for sex and love. These dynamics fashioned what we call our soul. Love and sex built human nature.

I've stood at the side of a few deathbeds. The last thoughts of my loved ones—be they man or woman, young or elderly—have always concerned two preoccupations: sex and people they love.

In the end, humans give in to love. *Homo sapiens* were designed by love for love. Falling in love is the biological purpose of human life.

The difference in men's and women's breeding strategies designs us to compete. But men's and women's shared interest in rearing a child through a long childhood designs men and women to cooperate. This exquisite tension between men's and women's desire to compete and cooperate makes us one of the horniest and most romantic mammals. It helped us breed each other for qualities we want in each other.

We did it for the family.

I thought writing this book would help me use my geekdom to get chicks. Instead it got me married. A million years of female choice caused the evolution of the husband instinct to evolve in male *Homo Sapiens*, despite the sperm factory in his pants.

Afterword

Crack open a cadaver's skull and take the brain out. You don't need to look at a human brain for very long to tell whether it's a male brain or a female brain. Men's and women's different jobs gave them different brains. Our species took advantage of these differences by specializing in different Pleistocene tasks. Now we understand why the other sex feels what it feels. If you want to find out how the other sex thinks, check out the next book in our series: *Tools Are from Men; Talk Is from Women: Why the Other Sex's Brain Is Weird*.

Notes

CHAPTER 1. The Sperm and Egg Problem

1. Trivers, R.L. 1972. "Parental investment and sexual selection." *Sexual Selection and the Descent of Man* ed. Campbell, B. Chicago: Aldine.136–179

2. Ridley, Mark. 1978. "Paternal care." *Animal Behavior* 26:904–932.

3. Eibl-Eibesfeldt, Ireanus. 1989. *Human Ethology*. New York: Aldine de Gruyter. 224–238.

4. Ridley, Matt. 1994. *The Red Queen: Sex and the Evolution of Human Nature*. New York: Macmillan. 171–244.

5. Kinsey, Alfred C. et al. 1948/1998. *Sexual Behavior in the Human Male*. Bloomington, IN: Indiana U. Press. 585, 587.

6. Kinsey, Alfred C. et al. 1953/1998. *Sexual Behavior in the Human Female*. Bloomington, IN: Indiana U. Press. 416.

CHAPTER 2. Female Promiscuity Controls the Size of Your Testicles

1. Short, R.V. 1979. "Sexual selection and its component parts, somatic and genital selection, as illustrated in man and great apes." *Advances in the Study of Behavior* 9:131–158.

2. Short, R.V. 1981. "Testis weight, body weight, and breeding systems in primates." *Nature* 293:55.

3. Baker, R. and Bellis, M.A. 1995. *Human Sperm Competition, Copulation, Masturbation, and Infidelity*. Chapman and Hall

4. Buss, David M. 1994. *The Evolution of Desire: Strategies in Human Mating*. New York: Basic Books. 130

CHAPTER 3. What Women Want

1. Sade, D.S. 1967. "Determinants of dominance in a group of free ranging rhesus monkeys." *Social Communication Among Primates* ed. Altmann, S.A. Chicago: University of Chicago Press:99–114.

2. Buss 1994. *Evolution of Desire*. 19–48

3. Elder, G.H. Jr. 1969. "Appearance and education in marriage mobility."

American Sociological Review. 344:519-533.

4. Taylor, P.A. & Glenn, N.D. 1976. "The utility of education and attractiveness for females' status attainment through marriage." *American Sociological Review.* 41:484-498.

5. Jackson, L.A. 1992. "Physical Appearance and Gender." *Sociobiological and Sociocultural Perspectives.* Albany: University of New York Press.

CHAPTER 4. Bodies and Resumes: What Makes Us Horny

1. Quirk, J. 2003. "Drunken frat boys and menopausal groupies." As yet unpublished in a peer-reviewed science journal.

CHAPTER 8. The Catfight Gene

1. Hurtado, A.M., & Hill, K.R. 1992. "Paternal effect on offspring survivorship among Ache and Hiwi hunter-gatherers: Implications for modeling pair-bond stability." *Father-Child Relations: Cultural and Biosocial Contexts* ed. Hewlett, Barry S. New York: Aldine de Gruyter:31-55.

2. Geary, David C. 1998. *Male, Female: The Evolution of Human Sex Differences.* Washington D.C.: American Psychological Association.

CHAPTER 9. The Jerk Gene

1. Le Boeuf, B. J., Petrinovich, L.F. 1974. "Elephant seals: Interspecific comparisons of vocal and reproductive behavior." *Mammalia.* 38:16-32.

2. Ellis, B.J. 1992. "The evolution of sexual attraction: Evaluative mechanisms in women." *The Adapted Mind: Evolutionary Psychology and The Generation of Culture.* eds Barkow, Cosmides, and Tooby. New York, NY: Oxford University Press. 267-288

3. Secord, P.F. 1982. "The origin and maintenance of social roles: The case of sex roles." *Personality, Roles, and Social Behavior.* eds. Ickes, W. and Knowles, E.S. New York: Springer:33-53.

4. Jobling, Mark A. 2001. "In the name of the father: surnames and genetics." *Trends In Genetics.* 176:353-7.

5. Buss, *Evolution of Desire.*

6. Ardener, E.W., et al. 1960. *Plantation and Village in the Cameroons.* London: Oxford University Press.

7. Betzig, L.L. 1989. "Causes of conjugal dissolution: A cross-cultural study." *Current Anthropology*. 30:654–676.

8. Frayser, Suzzane G. 1985. *Varieties of Sexual Experience: An Anthropological Perspective on Human Sexuality*. New Haven: HRAF Press. 258

CHAPTER 10. Bower Birds Teach Us How Art Evolved to Get the Groupie

1. Miller, Geoffrey. 2000. *The Mating Mind: How Sexual Choice Shaped the Evolution of Human Nature*. New York: Doubleday.

2. Darwin, Charles. 1871. *The Descent of Man and Selection in Relation to Sex*. London: John Murray. 342–343

CHAPTER 11. Male Promiscuity Decides Your Height

1. DiPietro, J.A. 1981. "Rough and tumble play: A function of gender." *Developmental Psychology*. 17:50–58.

2. Aldis, O. 1975. *Play-Fighting*. New York: Academic Press.

3. Whyte, M.K. 1978. "Cross-cultural codes dealing with the relative status of women." *Ethnology*. 17:211–37.

CHAPTER 12. Why Women Are Coy, Men Clueless

1. Alexander, R.D., and Noonan, K.M. 1979. "Concealment of ovulation, parental care, and human social evolution." *Evolutionary Biology and Human Social Behavior* eds. Chagnon, N.A. and Irons, W.G. Duxbury, Scituate: North Duxbury Press. 436–453.

CHAPTER 14. Darwinism: Survival of the Sexiest

1. Hrdy, Sarah Blaffer. 1999. *Mother Nature: A History of Mothers, Infants, and Natural Selection*. New York: Pantheon. 136.

2. Kaplan, Hilliard. 1994: "Evolutionary wealth flows theories of fertility: empirical tests and new models." *Population and Development Review*. 20(4)753–91

3. www.stevequayle.com/Giants/Africa/Giants.Africa1.html.

4. Gunther, John. 1955. *Inside Africa* New York: Harper & Bros.. 229, 685–6.

5. Kittler, Glenn D. 1961. *Let's Travel in the Congo*. Chicago: The Children's Press: 30.

CHAPTER 15. How Kindness Became Sexy
1. Miller, *Mating Mind*.

CHAPTER 17. Why We Are Fat
1. Burnham, Terry, & Phelan, Jay. 2000. *Mean Genes: From Sex to Money to Food: Taming Our Primal Instincts*. Cambridge, MA.: Perseus. 35-6

CHAPTER 18. Aqua-Ape: The Missing Link?
1. Morris, Desmond. 1967. *The Naked Ape*. New York: McGraw-Hill.
2. Hardy, A.C. 1960. "Was man more aquatic in the past?" *New Scientist.* 7:642-645.
3. For more info on the debate: www.absoluteastronomy.com/encyclopedia/a/aq/aquatic_ape_hypothesis.htm

CHAPTER 19. Why You Like Spielberg More than T. S. Eliot
1. MacLean, Paul D. 1990. *The Triune Brain in Evolution: Role in Paleo Cerebral Functions*. New York: Plenum.

CHAPTER 20. Let's Face It
1. Ekman, P. 1993. "Facial expression and emotion." *American Psychologist*, 48(4):384-392.
2. Ekman, P. 1994. "Strong evidence for universals in facial expression: A reply to Russell's mistaken critique." *Psychological Bulletin.* 115:268-287.
3. Ekman, Paul & Davidson, Richard J. (Eds.) 1994. *The Nature of Emotion: Fundamental Questions*. New York: Oxford University Press.
4. Ekman, P. & Friesen, W.V. 1975 *Unmasking the Face: A Guide to Recognizing Emotions from Facial Clues*. Englewood Cliffs: Prentice-Hall.
5. Lazarus, Richard S. 1991. *Emotion and Adaptation*. New York: Oxford University Press.

CHAPTER 21. Love Stinks
1. Wedekind, C. et al. 1995. "MHC-dependent mate preferences in humans." *Proceedings of the Royal Society of London* B:260, 245-249
2. Cowley, J.J. and Brooksbank, B.W.L. 1991. "Human exposure to puta-

tive pheromones and changes in aspects of social behavior." *The Journal of Steroid Biochemistry and Molecular Biology*. 39:647–659

3. Churchman, Deborah. Sept. 1992. "Ibex: King of the Mountain." *Ranger Rick*. 26:9:5–8.

CHAPTER 23. You Don't Have An Orgasm. An Orgasm Has You.

1. Grammer, Karl 1996. "The Human Mating Game: The Battle of the Sexes and the War of Signals." Paper presented at the Human Behavior and Evolution Society annual conference, Northwestern University, Evanston, IL.

2. Tutin, C.E.G. 1979. "Mating patterns and reproductive strategies in a community of wild chimpanzees (*Pan troglodytes schweinfurthii*)." *Behavioral Ecology and Sociobiology*. 6:29–38.

3. Baker and Bellis, 1995. *Human Sperm Competition*.

CHAPTER 24. Why Your Clitoris is Hard to Find

1. Miller, *Mating Mind*. 238–241

CHAPTER 25. March of the Penguin Prostitutes

1. Jones, S. 2003. *Y: The Descent of Men: Revealing the Mysteries of Maleness.* New York: Houghton Mifflin. 136–8

2. Buss, 1994. *Evolution of Desire*. 125–9

CHAPTER 26. Free Love Causes War

1. Hames, R.B. 1996. "Costs and benefits of monogamy and polygyny for Yanomamo women." *Ethology and Sociobiology*. 17:181–199.

2. Chisholm, J.S., and Burbank, V.K. 1991. "Monogamy and polygyny in southeast Arnhem Land: Male coercion and female choice." *Ethology and Sociobiology*. 12:291–313.

3. Dorjahn, V.R. 1958. "Fertility, polygyny, and their interrelations in Temne society." *American Anthropologist*. 60(5):838–860.

4. Daly, Martin. & Wilson, M. 1988 *Homicide*. Hawthorne, N.Y.: Aldine de Gruyter.

5. Nisbett, Richard E. & Cohen, D. 1996. *Culture of Honor: The Psychology*

of Violence in the South. Boulder: Westview Press.

CHAPTER 27. Bimbos and Cuckolds: What Makes Us Jealous

1. Greiling, H. and Buss, D.M. 2000. "Women's sexual strategies; the hidden dimension of EPM." *Personality and Individual Differences.* 28:929–963.

2. Glass, S.P. and Wright, T.L. 1992. "Justifications for extramarital relationships: the association between attitudes, behaviors, and gender." *Journal of Sex Research.* 29:361–387.

3. Buss, 1994. *Evolution of Desire.*

4. Grammer, K. 1992. "Variations on a theme: Age dependent mate selection in humans." *Behavioural and Brain Sciences.* 17-1:100-2.

5. Udry, J.R. & Ecklund, B.K. 1984. "Benefits of being attractive: Differential payoffs for men and women." *Psychological Reports.* 54:47–56.

6. Symons, Donald. 1979. *The Evolution of Human Sexuality.* New York: Oxford University Press.

7. Brown, Donald E. 1991. *Human Universals.* New York: McGraw-Hill.

CHAPTER 29. Dying For Sex

1. Rogers, A.R. 1994. "Evolution of time preference by natural selection." *The American Economic Review.* 84(3):460–481.

CHAPTER 30. When Your Wife Sleeps With Your Brother, and You're Okay with That

1. Emlen, S.T., et al. 1998. "Cuckoldry as a cost of polyandry in the sexrole reversed wattled jacana, *Jacana jacana.*" *Proceedings of the Royal Society of London, Series B* 265:2539–2364.

2. Jenni, D.A. 1974. "Evolution of polyandry in birds." *American Zoologist.* 14:129–144.

3. Goldizen, A.W., et al. 1998. "Variable mating patterns in Tasmanian Native Hens (*Gallinula mortierii*): Correlates of reproductive success." *Journal of Animal Ecology.* 67:307–317.

4. Goldizen, A.W., J.C. Buchan, D.A. Putland, A.R. Goldizen, and E.A. Krebs. (2000) "Patterns of mate-sharing in a population of Tasmanian Native Hens (*Gallinula mortierii*)." *Journal of Animal Ecology.* 142:40–47.

5. Krakauer, Alan H. March 2005. "Kin selection and cooperative courtship in wild turkeys" in *Nature* 434:69-72.

6. Check out the turkey film:

www.berkeley.edu/news/media/releases/2005/03/02_turkeys.shtml

CHAPTER 31. Broad Hips, Big Butts; Broad Shoulders, Big Diction

1. Seid, Roberta Pollack. 1989. *Never Too Thin: Why Women Are at War with Their Bodies*. New York: Prentice Hall Press.

2. Low, B.S., et al. 1987. "Human hips, breasts, and buttocks: Is fat deceptive?" *Ethology and Sociobiology*. 8:249-257.

3. Sobal, J. and Stunkard, A.J. 1989 "Socioeconomic status and obesity: a review of the literature." *Psychological Bulletin*. 105:260-275.

4. Brink, P.J. 1989. "The fattening room among the Annang of Nigeria." *Medical Anthropology*. 131-143

5. Singh, Devendra 1993. "Adaptive significance of waist-to-hip ratio and female attractiveness." *Journal of Personality and Social Psychology*. 65:181-190;293-307.

6. Singh, Devendra. 1995. "Female judgment of male attractiveness and desirability for relationships: role of waist-to-hip ratio and financial status." *Journal of Personality and Social Psychology*. 69:1089-1101.

7. Singh, Devendra and Luis, S. 1995. "Ethnic and Gender Consensus for the effect of waist-to-hip ratio on judgment of women's attractiveness." *Human Nature*. 6:51-65.

8. Wetsman, A. and Marlowe, F. 1999. "How universal are male waist-to-hip ratio preferences? Evidence from the Hazda of Tanzania." *Evolution and Human Behavior*. 20:219-228.

9. Tovee, M.J. et al. 1997. "Supermodels: stick insects or hourglasses?" *Lancet*. 350:1474-5.

10. Yu, Douglas et al. 1998. "Is beauty in the eye of the beholder?" *Nature*. 396:321-322.

11. Yu, D.W. & Shepard, G. H. 1999. "The mystery of female beauty: Reply." *Nature*. 399:216.

12. Miller, *Mating Mind*.

CHAPTER 32. Why Your Penis Is Easy to Find
1. Kirkpatrick, M. 1989. "Sexual selection. Is bigger always better?" in *Nature.* 337:116.
2. Miller, *Mating Mind.*
3. Stubbs, R.H. 1997. "Penis lengthening—A retrospective review of 300 consecutive cases." *Canadian Journal of Plastic Surgery.* 5(2):93-100.

CHAPTER 33. Two Genes for Two Types of Gay Guys
1. Hamer, D.H., et al. 1993. "A linkage between DNA markers on the X chromosome and male sexuality orientation." *Science.* 261:321-327.
2. Hu, S, et al. 1995. "Linkage between sexual orientation and chromosome Xq28 in males but not females." *Nature Genetics.* 11:248-256.
3. Rice, G., et al. 1999. "Male homosexuality: absence of linkage to microsatellite markers at Xq28." *Science.* 284:665-667.

CHAPTER 36. Homo *Homo sapiens*
1. Zhou, J.N., et al. 1995. "A sex difference in the human brain and its relation to transsexuality." *Nature* 378:68-70.
2. LeVay, S. 1991. "A difference in hypothalamic structure between heterosexual and homosexual men." *Science.* 253:1034-7.
3. LeVay, S. 1993. *The Sexual Brain.* Cambridge, MA: MIT Press.
4. LeVay, S.—personal communication

CHAPTER 38. Why Men Have Nipples
1. Meyer-Bahlburg, H.F.L., et al. 1995. "Prenatal estrogen and the development of homosexual orientation." *Developmental Psychology.* 31:12-21.
2. Reinisch, J.M. 1981. "Prenatal exposure to synthetic progestins increases potential for aggression in humans." *Science.* 211:1171-1173.
3. Berenbaum, S.A. and Hines, M. 1992. "Early androgens are related to childhood sex-typed toy preferences." *Psychological Science.* 3:203-206.
4. Berenbaum, S.A., et al. 1995 "Early hormones and sex differences in cognitive abilities." *Learning and Individual Differences.* 7:303-321.

CHAPTER 40. Falling in Love

1. Jankowiak, W.R., and Fisher, E.F. 1992. "A cross-cultural perspective on romantic love" *Ethnology*. 31:149-55.

In Case You Think I'm Full of It: Bibliography

Barkow, Jerome H., Cosmides, Leda and Tooby, John. (Eds.) 1992. *The Adapted Mind: Evolutionary Psychology and the Generation of Culture*. New York: Oxford University Press.

Bloom, Howard. 1995. *The Lucifer Principle: A Scientific Expedition into the Forces of History*. New York: Atlantic Monthly Press.

——2000. *Global Brain: The Evolution of Mass Mind from the Big Bang to the 21st Century*. New York: John Wiley & Sons, Inc.

Brown, Donald E. 1991. *Human Universals*. New York: McGraw-Hill.

Burnham, R., & Phelan, J., 2000. *Mean Genes: From Sex to Money to Food: Taming Our Primal Instincts*. Cambridge, MA: Perseus.

Buss, David M. 1994. *The Evolution of Desire: Strategies in Human Mating*. New York: Basic Books.

Cartwright, John. 2000. *Evolution and Human Behavior*. Cambridge, MA: MIT Press.

Darwin, Charles. 1871. *The Descent of Man and Selection in Relation to Sex*. London. John Murray.

Dawkins, Richard. 1976/1989. *The Selfish Gene* (new ed.) New York: Oxford University Press.

de Waal, Frans. 1998. *Chimpanzee Politics: Power and Sex among Apes*. (rev. ed.) Baltimore: John Hopkins University Press.

de Waal, Frans and Lanting, Frans. 1997. *Bonobo: The Forgotten Ape*. University of California Press.

Diamond, Jared. 1992. *The Third Chimpanzee: The Evolution and Future of the Human Animal*. New York: HarperCollins.

Dissanayake, Ellen. 1992. *Homo Aestheticus: Where Art Comes From and Why*. New York: Free Press

Fisher, Helen E. 1982. *The Sex Contract: The Evolution of Human Behavior*. William Morrow.

Geary, David C. 1998. *Male, Female: The Evolution of Human Sex Differences*. Washington D.C.: American Psychological Association.

Low, Bobbi. 1999. *Why Sex Matters: A Darwinian Look at Human Behavior*.

Princeton University Press.

Miller, Geoffrey. 2000. *The Mating Mind: How Sexual Choice Shaped the Evolution of Human Nature.* New York: Doubleday.

Morris, Desmond. 1967. *The Naked Ape.* New York: McGraw-Hill.

Pinker, Steven. 2002. *The Blank Slate: The Modern Denial of Human Nature.* New York: Viking

Ridley, Matt. 1994. *The Red Queen: Sex and the Evolution of Human Nature.* New York: Macmillan.

Wilson, Edward O. 1979. *On Human Nature.* New York: Bantam.

—1975/2000. *Sociobiology: The New Synthesis (25th anniversary ed.).* Cambridge, MA: Harvard University Press.

—1998. *Consilience: The Unity of Knowledge.* New York: Knopf.

Wright, Robert. 1994. *The Moral Animal: Evolutionary Psychology and Everyday Life.* New York: Pantheon.

Useless Index

People Who Deserve Acknowledgement but not Payment

The Meridian Gallery lets our San Francisco Writer's Workshop meet on their premises every week for free, and without that institution this book would suck.

To the genius scientific synthesizer, Howard Bloom, thank you for introducing me to Richard Curtis. Please stop writing better books than me.

My agent, Richard Curtis, thank you for tirelessly prodding me to do all the work.

My editor Lisa Clancy, thank you for your diligence and insight. John Douglas and Nancy Pines, thank you for your sharp eyes. My mistakes were Lisa's fault. Matt Bell, thanks for the enlightening critique. Keep your thoughts to yourself from now on.

To all the low-paid scientists who did the real labor, painstakingly assembling the minutiae of data and making it available to the public: Thanks, suckers.

Mom, I couldn't have done it without your nagging. This book should make up for all the times I embarrassed you in public.

About the Author

JOE QUIRK is a sperm-spreading author who evolved from monkey business to monogamy when he married. He lives in Northern California with his wife and two cats he would like to kill. He is the author of the novel *The Ultimate Rush*.